Medical and Surgical Emergencies for Students and Junior Doctors

FAYE HILL, SASH NOOR AND NEEL SHARMA

Foreword by
TIAGO VILLANUEVA
General Practitioner
Former BMJ Clegg Scholar
Past Editor of the Student BMJ

Radcliffe Publishing
London • New York

Radcliffe Publishing Ltd
St Mark's House
Shepherdess Walk
London N1 7LH
United Kingdom

www.radcliffehealth.com

British Library Cataloguing in Publication Data

A catalogue record for this book is available from the British Library.

ISBN-13: 978 184619 503 7

Typeset by Darkriver Design, Auckland, New Zealand
Printed and bound by Cadmus Communications, USA

Contents

Foreword

Whether it's in the hospital ward, the emergency department, the operating room or the GP practice, medical and surgical emergencies are always bound to happen. The management of such emergencies is both difficult and challenging, and can be quite daunting for medical students and junior doctors. Sound preparation is therefore key.

Faye Hill, Sash Noor and Neel Sharma have come up with a wonderful new resource that will help empower medical students and junior doctors to handle medical and surgical emergencies with increasing confidence. The concise, well-structured format makes the book useful at the point of care, as well as during revision prior to a ward round, a shift in the emergency department and, of course, both written and oral exams. It will also be of interest to doctors involved in educating medical students and junior doctors, who may find it a source of inspiration.

Dr Tiago Villanueva
General Practitioner
Former BMJ Clegg Scholar
Past Editor of the *Student BMJ*
October 2013

Preface

Despite completing numerous examinations at medical school, it is clearly apparent that both students and junior doctors have difficulty in managing acute medical and surgical situations. This is in part due to a lack of actual patient exposure and subsequent management during undergraduate and early postgraduate training.

This book aims to provide a comprehensive coverage of the common medical and surgical emergencies one is likely to face during student and junior doctor training. In addition, its usage of evidence-based practice ensures that it is relevant for today's practice.

We would like to point out that this text is by no means a replacement volume for acute emergencies but, rather, a handbook for ease of use on the wards. With regard to pharmaceutical management, we have aimed to include typical drugs prescribed for many cases but have avoided drug doses in the main. This is an area that is constantly changing and best practice relies on concurrent use of the *British National Formulary* and pharmaceutical guidelines at your designated hospital.

In addition, we are more than happy to answer any queries based on the material provided, so please feel free to contact us via Radcliffe Publishing at contact.us@radcliffepublishing.com. Furthermore, if readers feel strongly that certain key topics should be included, we are more than happy to construct additional material as part of Radcliffe's e-bulletins.

We sincerely hope you find this book useful and wish you all the success in your future careers.

Faye Hill
Sash Noor
Neel Sharma
October 2013

About the authors

Faye Hill graduated from The University of Manchester with a bachelor's degree in medicine. She is now studying for a Master of Science in Internal Medicine from The University of Edinburgh. Faye completed foundation training in Preston and is now an emergency medicine core trainee in Sheffield. She has an ongoing interest in medical education and volunteers as a problem-based learning tutor for undergraduates.

Sash Noor, after completing her bachelor's degree in medicine at The University of Manchester, completed her foundation years at Royal Preston Hospital. She is currently an emergency medicine core trainee in South Manchester, where she continues to be actively involved in undergraduate education.

Neel Sharma graduated from The University of Manchester with bachelor degrees in pharmacology and medicine. He also holds a Master of Science in Gastroenterology from Barts and The London School of Medicine and Dentistry. Neel undertook his foundation and core medical training in London and maintains a strong interest in medical education. He was appointed Clinical Lecturer at the Centre for Medical Education at Barts in 2011, and he previously held the position of Tutor at the Institute of Medical and Health Sciences Education, Li Ka Shing Faculty of Medicine, The University of Hong Kong, from 2012 to 2013. He is also a member of the Curriculum Development Team for the newly established Lee Kong Chian School of Medicine in Singapore.

Contributors

Dr Janet Ling
Core Medical Trainee, Singapore

Dr Kristian Skinner
Core Medical Trainee, Blackpool

I would like to dedicate this book to my boyfriend and my family, especially my mum, who lovingly and patiently support me through everything I do.

FH

I would like to dedicate this to my friends and family; thank you for all your love and support during the good times, and for even more love and support during the less than good!

SN

I would like to dedicate this book to my parents, Ravi and Anita, and my sister, Ravnita. Without their continued support and encouragement none of this would have truly been possible.

NS

MEDICINE

Chapter 1

GASTROENTEROLOGY

Clostridium difficile

Symptoms
➲ Watery diarrhoea, abdominal pain, fever

Signs
➲ Abdominal tenderness, fever, dehydration, rebound tenderness in cases of possible perforation

Differentials
➲ Crohn's disease
➲ Ulcerative colitis
➲ Diverticular disease
➲ Toxic megacolon
➲ Salmonella
➲ Shigella

How to investigate?
Investigations of choice include a full blood count, urea and electrolytes, C-reactive protein and serum lactate. Stools should of course be sent for screening of *C. difficile*. A colonoscopy or sigmoidoscopy can help to confirm the existence of pseudomembranous colitis, recognised as yellow-white plaques overlying oedematous mucosa.

How to manage?
The medical treatment of *C. difficile* relies upon 500 mg of metronidazole administered orally for 10 days in non-severe cases and 125 mg of vancomycin administered orally four times daily for 10 days in severe cases. An alternative to vancomycin is teicoplanin. When oral therapy is not possible, patients should be commenced on 500 mg of metronidazole administered intravenously for 10 days in non-severe cases. Metronidazole and intracolonic or nasogastric vancomycin is worthwhile in severe cases.

The decision to undertake surgery is based upon whether there is perforation of the colon and a worsening clinical state.

Upper gastrointestinal bleeding

Symptoms

⊃ Weakness, dizziness, fainting (syncope), coffee-ground vomit, black stool, indigestion, heartburn, abdominal pain, swallowing difficulties (dysphagia), weight loss

Signs

⊃ Haematemesis, melaena, haemodynamic instability such as hypotension, tachycardia, cool extremities, signs of chronic liver disease

Differentials

⊃ Abdominal aortic aneurysm
⊃ Peptic ulcer
⊃ Varices
⊃ Oesophageal or gastric malignancy
⊃ Oesophagitis or gastritis

How to investigate?

Patients presenting with an upper gastrointestinal bleed should undergo Glasgow–Blatchford and Rockall scoring.

Glasgow–Blatchford Score Criteria

Admission risk marker	Score component value
Blood urea (mmol/L)	
≥6·5 <8·0	2
≥8·0 <10·0	3
≥10·0 <25·0	4
≥25	6
Haemoglobin (g/dL) for men	
≥12.0 <13.0	1
≥10.0 <12.0	3
<10.0	6
Haemoglobin (g/dL) for women	
≥10.0 <12.0	1
<10.0	6

(*continued*)

Admission risk marker	Score component value
Systolic blood pressure (mmHg)	
100–109	1
90–99	2
<90	3
Other markers	
Pulse ≥100 (per minute)	1
Presentation with melaena	1
Presentation with syncope	2
Hepatic disease	2
Cardiac failure	2

A Glasgow–Blatchford score of 6 or more is associated with a 50% chance of requiring an intervention such as a transfusion, endoscopy or surgery.

Rockall Score Criteria

Variable	Scores				
	0	1	2	3	
Age (years)	<60	60–79	>80		Initial score
Shock	No shock	Tachycardia, pulse >100 beats per minute	Hypotension, SBP <100 mmHg		
Co-morbidity	No major co-morbidity		Cardiac failure, IHD, any major co-morbidity	Renal failure, liver failure, disseminated malignancy	
Diagnosis	Mallory-Weiss tear, no lesion identified and no stigmata of recent haemorrhage	All other diagnoses	Malignancy of upper GI tract		Additional criteria for full score
Major stigmata of recent haemorrhage	None, or dark spot only		Blood in upper GI tract, adherent clot, visible or spurting vessel		

Note: GI, gastrointestinal; IHD, ischaemic heart disease; SBP, systolic blood pressure

Patients with a pre-endoscopic Rockall score above 0 are associated with significant mortality and only those scoring 0 can be safely discharged. A full Rockall score of <3 is associated with 0.8% mortality, with a re-bleeding rate of 6.7%.

Investigations of choice include a full blood count, renal profile, liver function tests and coagulation screen, in addition to a 'group and save' and crossmatch.

How to manage?

Platelets should be transfused for those patients with a platelet count of less than 50×10^9/L and who are actively bleeding. Fresh frozen plasma is used in cases where the fibrinogen level is <1 g/L or the prothrombin time or activated partial thromboplastin time is more than 1.5 times normal. Patients receiving warfarin who are actively bleeding should be given prothrombin complex.

Endoscopy is key and should be offered within 24 hours of presentation.

Non-variceal bleeds are best managed through an array of methods such as clips, adrenaline, thermal means, fibrin or thrombin. Proton pump inhibitors should be given to patients with evidence of non-variceal bleeding at time of endoscopy.

Variceal bleeds at presentation should be treated with terlipressin. Oesophageal varices are appropriately managed with band ligation and, if unsuccessful, with transjugular intrahepatic portosystemic shunting. Gastric varices are most commonly treated with N-butyl-2 cyanoacrylate.

Patients receiving drugs such as aspirin, clopidogrel and non-steroidal anti-inflammatory drugs should be assessed for risk of bleeding if continuing with such treatment.

Lower gastrointestinal bleeding

Symptoms
⊃ Blood/mucus in stool, abdominal pain, diarrhoea, fainting (syncope), dehydration, weight loss, fever

Signs
⊃ Blood on rectal examination, haemodynamic instability, abdominal tenderness

Differentials
⊃ Inflammatory bowel disease
⊃ Haemorrhoids
⊃ Anal fissure
⊃ Malignancy
⊃ Arteriovenous malformation

- Ischaemic colitis
- Diverticular disease
- Radiation proctitis
- Meckel's diverticulum
- Intussusception

How to investigate?

Blood investigations are of course essential, including a full blood count, urea and electrolytes, coagulation profile, 'group and save' and crossmatch. Further investigations include a colonoscopy, an abdominal CT scan or computed tomography angiography.

How to manage?

Colonoscopic haemostasis is a worthwhile intervention in those patients with bleeding secondary to diverticular disease or after a polypectomy. If bleeding continues then an angiographic transarterial embolisation is preferred or surgical excision.

Acute liver failure

Symptoms
- Yellow discolouration of skin and eyes (jaundice), lethargy, confusion, somnolence, abdominal pain

Signs
- Jaundice, abdominal tenderness, ascites, haemodynamic instability

Differentials
- Decompensated cirrhosis
- Alcoholic hepatitis
- Autoimmune hepatitis
- Eclampsia
- Sepsis

How to investigate?
Blood investigations of choice include a full blood count, renal profile including magnesium and phosphate, liver function tests, C-reactive protein and coagulation screen.

Lactate measurement is also key, as well as a serum paracetamol level, ammonia level and a toxicology screen. A hepatitis screen, ceruloplasmin level and autoimmune profile are also worthwhile.

Imaging is often employed and relies on the use of abdominal ultrasound plus or minus computed tomography.

How to manage?

Management is dependent on the grade of encephalopathy. A CT brain scan should be performed to exclude intracranial pathology and the presence of oedema. Lactulose has been shown to be merited in such patients. Patients with grade III or IV encephalopathy should ideally be intubated, with the use of mannitol for severe elevation of intracranial pressure or herniation. Antibiotics as per hospital protocol should be prescribed to reduce risk of sepsis.

Patients with evidence of coagulopathy should be treated with vitamin K with fresh frozen plasma for those who are actively bleeding. Platelet transfusion is instigated in cases where the count is <10 000 mm³. Such patients are at risk of stress ulceration and should be prescribed a proton pump inhibitor.

In cases of ensuing renal failure and worsening haemodynamics, patients will benefit from pressor support as well as haemodialysis.

Acute inflammatory bowel disease

Symptoms
- ⊃ Abdominal pain, diarrhoea or constipation, mucus/blood in stool, weight loss, fever, urgency, nausea or vomiting

Signs
- ⊃ Fever, tachycardia, hypotension, abdominal mass, perianal fissure, fistulas, iritis, episcleritis, joint swelling, erythema nodosum, pyoderma gangrenosum

Differentials
- ⊃ Amoebiasis
- ⊃ Appendicitis
- ⊃ Coeliac disease
- ⊃ *Clostridium difficile*
- ⊃ Cytomegalovirus
- ⊃ Diverticulitis
- ⊃ Gastroenteritis
- ⊃ Giardia
- ⊃ Intestinal radiation-induced injury

How to investigate?

Blood investigations of choice include a full blood count, haematinics, urea and electrolytes, C-reactive protein and stool for microscopy, culture and sensitivity as well as *C. difficile*. A full colonoscopy is rarely warranted in the acute phase because of the risk of perforation, and patients typically benefit from a flexible sigmoidoscopy. An abdominal and chest X-ray helps to exclude toxic megacolon and perforation, respectively. Further imaging in the form of a CT scan plus or minus an MRI may help to determine the presence of abscess formation.

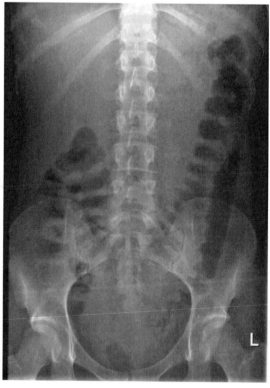

Abdominal X-ray demonstrating thickening of the descending and sigmoid colon, in keeping with active colitis

How to manage?

With regard to Crohn's disease, initial treatment relies upon the use of intravenous steroids – namely, hydrocortisone 100 mg four times daily. These are typically continued for 3–5 days with a view to converting to oral prednisolone, which is then gradually tapered according to clinical response. For those with steroid refractory disease, treatment relies upon azathioprine, 6 mercaptopurine (6-MP), methotrexate and anti-tumour necrosis factor-alpha therapy such as infliximab. Surgical intervention is paramount in cases of refractory treatment and worsening severity.

In acute cases of ulcerative colitis, it is important to gauge severity, courtesy of the Truelove and Witts' criteria.

Activity	Mild	Moderate	Severe
Number of bloody stools per day	<4	4-6	>6
Temperature (°C)	Afebrile	Intermediate	>37.8
Heart rate (beats per minute)	Normal	Intermediate	>90
Haemoglobin (g/dL)	>11	10.5-11	<10.5
Erythrocyte sedimentation rate (mm/hour)	<20	20-30	>30

Again intravenous hydrocortisone is employed for up to 5 days. Patients should be considered for intravenous ciclosporin plus or minus infliximab or a colectomy in view of worsening clinical condition by at least day three.

All patients in general should be commenced on subcutaneous heparin in view of the risk of thromboembolism and should have appropriate fluid and electrolyte resuscitation.

It is important to always appreciate the risk of toxic megacolon in acute colitis (diameter >5.5 cm) and the need for surgical intervention in such cases.

Acute pancreatitis

Symptoms
⊃ Abdominal pain epigastric in nature and radiating to the back, nausea, vomiting, diarrhoea, loss of appetite

Signs
⊃ Fever, tachycardia, abdominal tenderness, guarding, Cullen's sign (blue discolouration around umbilicus), Grey Turner's sign (red-brown discolouration of flanks), Purtscher's retinopathy

Differentials
⊃ Acute mesenteric ischaemia
⊃ Cholangitis

- Cholecystitis
- Chronic pancreatitis
- Colonic cancer
- Gastroenteritis
- Peptic ulcer
- Gastric and pancreatic cancer
- Pancreatic pseudocyst

How to investigate?

Investigations of choice include a serum amylase, lipase and CRP. Liver function tests are also useful in order to exclude pancreatitis secondary to gallstones. In order to ascertain aetiology, a serum cholesterol and lipid profile should be requested. In view of the Glasgow severity criteria, white blood cell count, serum glucose, lactate dehydrogenase, calcium, albumin, urea and an arterial blood gas should be performed.

- Age >55 years
- Serum albumin <32 g/L
- Arterial pO_2 (partial pressure of oxygen) on room air <8 kPa
- Serum calcium <2 mmol/L
- Blood glucose >10.0 mmol/L
- Serum lactate dehydrogenase >600 units/L
- Serum urea nitrogen >16 mmol/L
- White blood cell count >15 × 10^9/L
- Serum AST >200 iU/L

A score >2 implies a high likelihood of severe pancreatitis.

Imaging in terms of computed tomography is preferred over ultrasound, with severity of acute pancreatitis being determined utilising the following grading system.

Computed Tomography (CT) Grading of Severity

CT grade	
(A) Normal pancreas	0
(B) Oedematous pancreatitis	1
(C) B plus mild extrapancreatic changes	2
(D) Severe extrapancreatic changes including one fluid collection	3
(E) Multiple or extensive extrapancreatic collections	4
Necrosis	
None	0
<One third	2
>One third, <one half	4
>Half	6

CT severity index = CT grade + necrosis score

	Complications
0–3	8%
4–6	35%
7–10	92%
	Deaths
0–3	3%
4–6	6%
7–10	17%

Modified from the International Association of Pancreatology guidelines (Uhl, Warshaw, Imrie, *et al.* 2002) and based on Balthazar and colleagues (Balthazar, Freeny, van Sonnenberg 1994).

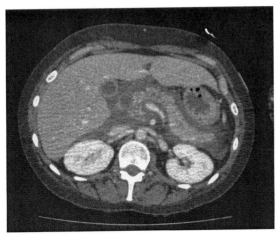

Abdominal CT scan demonstrating evidence of free fluid, gallstones and inflammatory changes in the pancreas, in keeping with acute pancreatitis

How to manage?

Antibiotic use is not so clear-cut with regard to management. If utilised, antibiotics of choice include ciprofloxacin, metronidazole and imipenem and should be continued for at least 14 days. Nutritional support should be provided in the form of enteral feeding, primarily via a nasogastric tube. For those patients with gallstone-related pancreatitis, an endoscopic retrograde cholangiopancreatogram should be performed. Following an acute attack, definitive treatment should be taken in the form of a cholecystectomy.

Gastroenteritis

Symptoms

⊃ Diarrhoea, blood and mucus in stool, vomiting, abdominal pain, fever, headache, muscle aches

Signs

⊃ Dehydration, blood or mucus per rectum, abdominal tenderness

Differentials

⊃ Appendicitis
⊃ Haemolytic uraemic syndrome
⊃ Inflammatory bowel disease
⊃ Small or large bowel obstruction

How to investigate?

Patients should undergo a full blood count, urea and electrolytes, C-reactive protein, stool microscopy, culture and sensitivity as well as ova, cysts and parasites. In cases of significant abdominal discomfort, patients may benefit from abdominal CT scanning. In cases where diarrhoea is persistent, a sigmoidoscopy may be warranted.

How to manage?

Management relies on the use of oral but more appropriately intravenous fluid replacement, typically with dextrose and saline. Depending on the cause, antibiotic therapies are instigated. *Escherichia coli,* Shigella and Salmonella can be suitably managed with ciprofloxacin. Campylobacter can be treated with erythromycin, and metronidazole for Giardia or Entamoeba. Antidiarrhoeals are best avoided but anti-emetics can be utilised for the relief of nausea and vomiting.

Chapter 2

RESPIRATORY

Pneumonia

Symptoms
⊃ Chest pain, shortness of breath (dyspnoea), haemoptysis, cough, sputum, fevers, diarrhoea in atypical cases such as Legionella

Signs
⊃ Fever, tachypnoea, accessory muscle use, tachycardia, cyanosis, confusion, crepitations, tracheal deviation, dullness to percussion

Differentials
⊃ Asthma
⊃ Bronchiectasis
⊃ Chronic obstructive pulmonary disease
⊃ Lung abscess
⊃ Respiratory failure

How to investigate?
A full blood count, urea and electrolytes, C-reactive protein and liver function tests are important in patients presenting with pneumonia. Sputum microscopy assessment is key, and should also be screened for *Mycobacterium tuberculosis*. A urinary screen is particularly important to screen for Legionella, pneumococcal and mycoplasma pneumonia. Blood cultures should also be requested ideally before antibiotics are started.

How to manage?
Such patients require appropriate oxygenation with a pO_2 aim of >8 kPa, and oxygen saturations between 94% and 98%. In view of sepsis, fluid resuscitation is paramount. As patients are likely to be immobile, venous thromboprophylaxis is key, with low-molecular-weight heparin. The initial chest X-ray should be repeated within 3 days if there has been no improvement in the clinical picture. Antibiotics are of course the mainstay form of treatment and are prescribed in accordance with the CURB-65 criteria (confusion, urea >7 mmol/L, respiratory rate >30 breaths/min, BP systolic <90 mmHg and/or diastolic <60 mmHg, age >65).
⊃ Low severity, CURB-65 0–1: amoxicillin
⊃ Moderate severity, CURB-65 2: amoxicillin plus clarithromycin, or benzylpenicillin plus clarithromycin
⊃ High severity, CURB-65 3–5: co-amoxiclav plus clarithromycin, typically intravenously

Antibiotics are typically continued for up to 7 days in low- or moderate-severity cases and for up to 7–10 days for high severity.

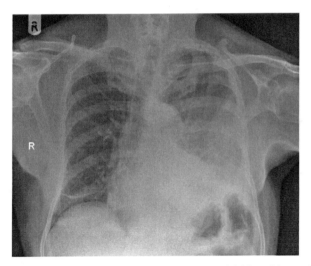

Chest X-ray demonstrating evidence of right lower zone atelectasis with left lower lobe consolidation and a left-sided pleural effusion

Asthma

Symptoms
⮞ Wheeze, cough, chest tightness, shortness of breath

Signs
⮞ Inability to communicate in sentences, wheeze, accessory muscle use, tachycardia, tachypnoea

Differentials
⮞ Aspergillosis
⮞ Bronchiectasis
⮞ Chronic obstructive pulmonary disease
⮞ Gastro-oesophageal reflux disease
⮞ Pulmonary embolism
⮞ Sarcoidosis

How to investigate?

Patients should undergo a full blood count, urea and electrolytes, C-reactive protein, and peak expiratory flow (PEF) rate measurement, in addition to a chest X-ray and an arterial blood gas. A raised blood eosinophil count may be observed.

How to manage?

Severity assessment must be undertaken for patients with acute asthma.

- ⇨ Moderate exacerbation: increasing symptoms, PEF >50%–75 % predicted, no features of acute severe asthma
- ⇨ Acute exacerbation: PEF 33%–50% best or predicted, respiratory rate of >25 breaths per minute, heart rate >110 beats per minute, inability to complete sentences in one breath
- ⇨ Life-threatening: PEF <33% predicted; SpO_2 (saturation of peripheral oxygen) <92%, pO_2 <8 kPa, normal pCO_2 (partial pressure of carbon dioxide), silent chest, cyanosis, poor respiratory effort, arrhythmias, exhaustion
- ⇨ Near fatal: raised pCO_2, need for mechanical ventilation.

Oxygen therapy is employed to ensure a SpO_2 of 94%–98%. High-dose inhaled beta 2 agonists should be given in nebulised form in addition to nebulised ipratropium bromide. Steroids should be prescribed, typically 40 mg daily for at least 5 days. Intravenous magnesium sulphate should be commenced at 1.2–2 g infusion over 20 minutes.

It is important to continually monitor such cases with a plan to refer to intensive care if patients meet the following criteria:

- ⇨ need for ventilatory support
- ⇨ deteriorating PEF
- ⇨ worsening hypoxia
- ⇨ hypercapnia
- ⇨ worsening respiratory acidosis
- ⇨ altered conscious state
- ⇨ respiratory arrest.

Chronic obstructive pulmonary disease

Symptoms

➲ Cough, sputum production, shortness of breath, wheeze

Signs

➲ Hyperinflation of chest, wheeze, hyper-resonance on percussion, accessory muscle use, cyanosis, pursed lip breathing

Differentials

➲ Emphysema
➲ Bronchitis
➲ Alpha 1-antitrypsin deficiency
➲ Pulmonary embolism

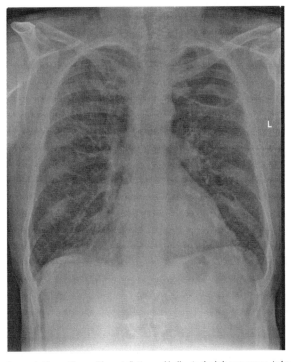

Chest X-ray demonstrating evidence of hyperinflation and bullae in the left upper zone, in keeping with chronic obstructive pulmonary disease

How to investigate?

Patients with a suspected acute exacerbation of chronic obstructive pulmonary disease should undergo an arterial blood gas, chest X-ray and ECG. Blood investigations include a full blood count, urea and electrolytes, C-reactive protein and blood cultures. Sputum should also be sent for microscopy, culture and sensitivity. If the patient is on theophylline, a theophylline level should be taken at admission.

How to manage?

Such patients should be treated with nebulised bronchodilators and in cases of purulent sputum production and chest X-ray consolidation, antibiotics such as aminopenicillin, a macrolide or tetracycline. Prednisolone 30 mg should be given daily for 7–14 days. Oxygen therapy should be commenced and monitored accordingly, with a saturation aim between the range of 88% and 92%. Intravenous theophyllines can be commenced if response to bronchodilator therapy is poor.

Non-invasive ventilation should be considered for patients who are slow to wean from invasive ventilation and for those with hypercapnic ventilatory failure. Doxapram is an alternative to non-invasive ventilation.

Patients should undergo regular arterial blood gas measurement and symptom assessment.

Acute respiratory distress syndrome

(PaO_2/FiO_2 ratio less than 200 mmHg and pulmonary capillary wedge pressure lower than 18 mmHg)

Symptoms
⊃ Dyspnoea, anxiety, agitation

Signs
⊃ Tachypnoea, tachycardia, hypotension, cyanosis, crepitations (and signs of underlying cause)

Differentials
⊃ Hypersensitivity pneumonitis
⊃ Pneumonia
⊃ Respiratory failure
⊃ Septic shock

How to investigate?

An arterial blood gas is an essential investigation of choice. B-type natriuretic peptide levels and an echocardiogram should be requested to exclude cardiogenic pulmonary oedema. Additional blood investigations include a full blood count, urea and electrolytes, liver function tests and C-reactive protein. A chest X-ray plus or minus a CT scan is an essential imaging test. A bronchoscopy may help to exclude the presence of infection, alveolar haemorrhage or acute eosinophilic pneumonia.

How to manage?

The mainstay form of treatment in such cases is supportive with treatment of the underlying cause. Supportive measures include prevention of deep vein thrombosis and pressure ulcers. The head of the bed should be maintained at a 30-degree angle to reduce the risk of a hospital-acquired pneumonia.

Patients should all be managed with positive pressure ventilation with supplemental oxygen and positive end-expiratory pressure. Research also demonstrates a potential benefit in prone positioning to enhance oxygenation in patients who are refractory to conventional treatment. The use of corticosteroids may also help to enhance gas exchange and haemodynamics. Nitric oxide has been shown to improve oxygenation and pulmonary vascular resistance.

Respiratory failure

Symptoms
- ➲ Dyspnoea, chest pain, shortness of breath when lying flat (orthopnoea)

Signs
- ➲ Hypoxia, asterixis in view of hypercapnia, tachycardia, cyanosis, dyspnoea, confusion, seizures, crepitations

Differentials
- ➲ Acute respiratory distress syndrome
- ➲ Asthma
- ➲ Cardiogenic shock
- ➲ Cor pulmonale
- ➲ Myocardial infarction
- ➲ Pneumonia
- ➲ Pneumothorax
- ➲ Pulmonary oedema

- Pulmonary embolism
- Pulmonary fibrosis

How to investigate?

Investigations of choice include a full blood count, urea and electrolytes and C-reactive protein. An arterial blood gas is essential, of course, to determine severity extent and the existence of type I or II respiratory failure. Additional investigations of choice include a chest X-ray, an echocardiogram and pulmonary function tests.

How to manage?

Such patients require appropriate airway stabilisation, assessment of oxygenation and haemodynamic stability with treatment of the underlying disease. These patients often require high-dependency or intensive care support. Studies have shown that the use of extracorporeal membrane oxygenation is positively beneficial in patients with evidence of hypercapnia and a pH <7.2.

Mechanical ventilation allows for an increase in pO_2 and a reduction in pCO_2. The general principle involves the use of positive pressure ventilation. From a medical perspective, drug therapies in the form of diuretics, nitrates, analgesia and inotropes are all required in cases of acute pulmonary oedema.

Pulmonary embolism

Symptoms
- Shortness of breath, pleuritic chest pain

Signs
- Dyspnoea, hypoxia, crepitations, tachycardia, cyanosis

Differentials
- Acute coronary syndrome
- Acute respiratory distress syndrome
- Cardiogenic shock
- Chronic obstructive pulmonary disease
- Congestive cardiac failure
- Fat embolism
- Pneumothorax
- Pulmonary oedema
- Pulmonary hypertension

- Myocardial infarction
- Cardiac tamponade

How to investigate?

Blood investigations, predominantly a D-dimer, should be performed following assessment of clinical probability and ideally in those with high clinical probability. From an imaging perspective, a CT pulmonary angiogram is the recommended imaging of choice in cases of non-massive and massive pulmonary embolism (PE). Isotope lung scanning is considered in cases of a normal chest X-ray in patients with no significant cardiopulmonary disease.

How to manage?

Patients with a working diagnosis of PE should be thrombolysed as a first-line treatment in cases of massive PE, with a 50 mg alteplase bolus. Prior to imaging, heparin should be given to patients with intermediate or high clinical probability. Unfractionated heparin should be considered as a first bolus dose, in cases of massive PE or where rapid reversal of effect is needed. Otherwise, as an alternative, low-molecular-weight heparin should be considered. Oral anticoagulation should be commenced once a PE has been confirmed. The target range of the international normalised ratio should be between 2 and 3, and once achieved, heparin can be ceased. The duration of treatment of oral anticoagulation is 4–6 weeks for temporary risk factors, 3 months for first idiopathic cases and at least 6 months in all other cases.

Pneumothorax

Symptoms
- Chest pain, shortness of breath

Signs
- Tachypnoea, asymmetrical lung expansion, absent air entry, hyper-resonance on percussion, tracheal shift to contralateral side, tachycardia, hypotension

Differentials
- Acute respiratory distress syndrome
- Oesophageal rupture
- Myocardial infarction
- Cardiac tamponade
- Pulmonary embolism

How to investigate?

Patients should undergo an arterial blood gas and an erect chest X-ray during inspiration for the initial diagnosis. A CT scan can be undertaken to aid detection of small pneumothoraces and for size estimation.

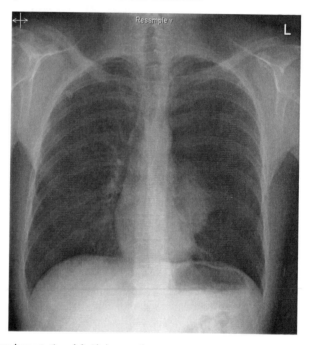

Chest X-ray demonstrating a left-sided pneumothorax

How to manage?

Management for a primary spontaneous pneumothorax depends on clinical assessment. For those with a small primary spontaneous pneumothorax without significant shortness of breath, observation is recommended. Those who are symptomatic with a pneumothorax ≥2 cm should undergo needle aspiration with a 16–18 G cannula. If unsuccessful, a chest drain should be inserted, typically size 8–14 Fr.

Patients with a secondary pneumothorax between 1 and 2 cm in size should undergo needle aspiration. Those greater than 2 cm should be selected for chest drain insertion. High-flow oxygen is recommended in these cases.

The use of chemical pleurodesis is advised in cases of difficult or recurrent pneumothoraces. From a surgical perspective, cases of persistent air leak or failure of lung expansion should be referred for thoracic input for open thoracotomy or video-assisted thoracic surgery.

Pleural effusion

Symptoms
- ⊃ Dyspnoea, cough, chest pain, shortness of breath lying flat (orthopnoea), night sweats, fever, haemoptysis, weight loss, sputum production

Signs
- ⊃ Dullness to percussion, reduced chest expansion, tracheal shift away from the effusion, reduced breath sounds

Differentials
- ⊃ Pulmonary oedema
- ⊃ Congestive cardiac failure
- ⊃ Lung malignancy
- ⊃ Oesophageal rupture
- ⊃ Pancreatitis

How to investigate?

Patients with a suspected pleural effusion should undergo a posteroanterior chest X-ray. Aspiration via ultrasound guidance is recommended typically with a 21 G needle. Fluid should be sent for protein, lactate dehydrogenase (LDH), Gram stain, cytology and microscopy, culture and sensitivity. It is important to assess whether the effusion is a transudate or exudate and this is easily achieved through Light's criteria

Light's criteria for an exudative effusion:
- ⊃ pleural fluid protein to serum protein ratio >0.5
- ⊃ pleural fluid LDH to serum LDH ratio >0.6
- ⊃ pleural fluid LDH greater than $\frac{2}{3}$ × serum LDH upper limit of normal.

The effusion should undergo pH testing, with a pH less than 7.2 indicating an empyema requiring drainage. Other investigations of choice include a CT scan in cases of undiagnosed exudative pleural effusions and to help distinguish malignant from benign pleural thickening. A percutaneous pleural biopsy is useful in investigating an undiagnosed effusion where malignancy is suspected. A thoracoscopy can be undertaken in cases of exudative pleural effusions where an aspiration is inconclusive and malignancy is suspected.

How to manage?

The general rule of thumb is treatment of the underlying cause and if the patient is symptomatic they should undergo chest drain insertion.

Chapter 3

RENAL

Acute renal failure or acute kidney injury

Symptoms

➲ Low urine output (oliguria), failure to produce urine (anuria), thirst, dizziness, confusion, blood in urine, fever, rash, joint pain, urinary urgency, urinary hesitancy, abdominal pain, muscle weakness, sensory loss

Signs

➲ Livedo reticularis, signs secondary to diabetes mellitus or hypertension, hearing loss in cases of aminoglycoside toxicity, pericardial rub in cases of uraemic pericarditis, abdominal tenderness, crepitations in cases of Goodpasture's syndrome or Wegener's granulomatosis

Differentials

➲ Acute tubular necrosis
➲ Acute glomerulonephritis
➲ Chronic renal failure
➲ Haemolytic uraemic syndrome

How to investigate?

Patients with acute renal failure or acute kidney injury should undergo blood investigations namely a full blood count, urea and electrolytes and C-reactive protein. Urine and bloods should be sent for culture if infection is suspected. Renal immunology should be requested – namely, serum ANA, ANCA, anti-double-stranded DNA and anti-GBM. Urine electrolytes and osmolality should be requested in addition to a chest X-ray, an ECG (in cases of hyperkalaemia) and a renal ultrasound scan ideally within 24 hours of presentation, plus or minus renal biopsy. With regard to urinary electrolytes, in pre-renal failure there is typically increased urinary sodium reabsorption and increased urinary urea absorption with low urine sodium concentrations.

How to manage?

Patients with acute renal failure or acute kidney injury should be appropriately fluid resuscitated according to volume status, typically with 0.9% sodium chloride. Patient medication should be reviewed to ensure any nephrotoxic drugs are ceased and vital drugs should be dosed in accordance with altered renal kinetics. Nutritional support is key, and patients should receive 25–35 kcal/kg/day. The decision to start renal replacement therapy is governed by the following criteria:

- ⮑ Biochemical indications:
  - refractory hyperkalaemia >6.5 mmol/L
  - serum urea >27 mmol/L
  - refractory metabolic acidosis pH <7.15
  - refractory electrolyte abnormalities:
    - — hyponatraemia, hypernatraemia or hypercalcaemia
    - — tumour lysis syndrome with hyperuricaemia and hyperphosphataemia
    - — urea cycle defects, and organic acidurias resulting in hyperammonaemia
- ⮑ Clinical indications:
  - urine output <0.3 mL/kg for 24 hours or absolute anuria for 12 hours
  - acute kidney injury with multiple organ failure
  - refractory volume overload
  - end-organ involvement: pericarditis, encephalopathy, neuropathy, myopathy, uraemic bleeding
  - creation of intravascular space for plasma and other blood product infusions and nutrition
  - severe poisoning or drug overdose
  - severe hypothermia or hyperthermia

Hyponatraemia

Symptoms
- ⮑ Nausea, headache, confusion, fits

Signs
- ⮑ Hypotension, tachycardia, dehydration

Differentials
- ⮑ Adrenal crisis
- ⮑ Alcohol excess
- ⮑ Cirrhosis
- ⮑ Hypothyroidism
- ⮑ Heart failure

How to investigate?
Investigations of choice include a urine osmolality, serum osmolality, urinary sodium concentration, thyroid function tests and serum cortisol. Useful imaging may include a CT head scan and chest X-ray.

How to manage?

In cases of hyponatraemia in patients who are hypervolaemic, the treatment of choice is salt and fluid restriction plus loop diuretic use. In hypovolaemic cases, saline replacement is required, and in euvolaemic cases fluid restriction is the treatment of choice. It is important to note that in all cases, treatment of the underlying cause is key. One must also be careful not to induce osmotic demyelination secondary to over-rapid correction of sodium.

From a pharmacological perspective, individuals with SIADH (syndrome of inappropriate antidiuretic hormone secretion – elevated urine osmolality and low plasma osmolality) are best managed with demeclocycline. In addition, vaptans and arginine vasopressin receptor antagonists have been utilised in the management of euvolaemic and hypervolaemic hyponatraemia.

Hyperkalaemia

Symptoms
⮞ Chest pain, weakness, numbness, palpitations

Signs
⮞ Cardiac dysrhythmia, diminished tendon reflexes, limb weakness

Differentials
⮞ Hypocalcaemia
⮞ Acute renal failure

How to investigate?

Investigations of choice include a full blood count, urea and electrolytes including serum calcium, urinalysis in cases of renal insufficiency and an ECG.

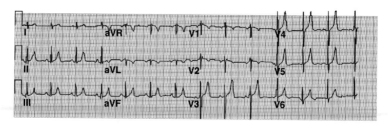

ECG demonstrating evidence of hyperkalaemia

How to manage?
Hyperkalaemia is a medical emergency and requires appropriate patient assessment. The treatment of hyperkalaemia involves calcium gluconate (cardio-protective), insulin–dextrose, salbutamol nebulisers and calcium resonium. The underlying cause should be sought and managed accordingly.

Hypercalcaemia

Symptoms
- Nausea, vomiting, confusion, abdominal pain, constipation, low mood, weakness, increased thirst and urinary frequency, headache

Signs
- Abdominal tenderness, muscle weakness, hyper-reflexia, fasciculations

Differentials
- Sarcoidosis
- Malignancy
- Hyperparathyroidism
- Tuberculosis

How to investigate?
Patients should undergo a full blood count, urea and electrolytes, serum parathyroid hormone, phosphate and vitamin D measurement. Imaging is worthwhile in cases of hypercalcaemia and suspected malignancy.

How to manage?
Management relies on treatment of the underlying cause, with a focus on rapid fluid resuscitation, use of loop diuretics and bisphosphonate therapies such as pamindronate.

Chapter 4

NEUROLOGY

Cord compression

Symptoms
- ➲ Back pain, stiffness, limb weakness, pins and needles, bladder or bowel dysfunction (constipation, urinary hesitancy, retention, incontinence)

Signs
- ➲ Spasticity, hyper-reflexia, loss of pinprick sensation, temperature, joint position and vibration

Differentials
- ➲ Transverse myelitis
- ➲ Multiple sclerosis
- ➲ Peripheral neuropathy

How to investigate?

The primary investigations of choice are typically imaging based. An MRI or CT scan of the spine is essential, with a standard spinal X-ray being less valuable. A CT myelograph may demonstrate an hourglass-type pattern of the contrast medium in such cases. Blood investigations should be requested, such as a full blood count and C-reactive protein to exclude infection, as well as blood cultures in the case of a suspected abscess, discitis or osteomyelitis.

How to manage?

First-line treatment involves immobilisation and urgent neurosurgical intervention. High-dose steroids have been shown to be of benefit, particularly in cases of malignancy, to help with pain relief and reduction of tumour-associated oedema. In cases of an epidural abscess, surgery in addition to antibiotic therapy, usually in the form of vancomycin, metronidazole and cefotaxime, is required.

Stroke

Symptoms
- ➲ Weakness, loss of sensation, visual loss, speech disturbance, unsteady gait, headache

Signs
- ➲ Hemiparesis, hemisensory deficit, visual field defects, diplopia, dysarthria, ataxia, vertigo, aphasia, atrial fibrillation, carotid bruits, hypertension

Differentials
- Brain abscess
- Brain neoplasm
- Subarachnoid haemorrhage
- Transient ischaemic attack
- Encephalitis
- Migraine
- Meningitis
- Subdural haematoma

How to investigate?

Blood investigations can help to determine cause such as evidence of polycythae-mia, thrombocytosis, thrombocytopenia or deranged coagulation. Brain imaging in the form of a CT scan or an MRI should be performed in the following cases:
- indications for thrombolysis or early anticoagulation treatment
- on anticoagulant treatment
- a known bleeding tendency
- a depressed level of consciousness (Glasgow Coma Scale score <13)
- unexplained progressive or fluctuating symptoms
- papilloedema, neck stiffness or fever
- severe headache at onset of stroke symptoms.

Additional imaging modalities include transcranial Doppler ultrasound, and an echocardiogram to exclude cardiogenic embolism should be instigated.

How to manage?

Thrombolysis with alteplase is indicated in cases of ischaemic stroke within 3 hours of symptom onset. Blood pressure monitoring is essential, with a target aim of 185/110 mmHg. Anti-hypertensive treatment should be given if there is a hypertensive emergency with one or more of the following:
- hypertensive encephalopathy
- hypertensive nephropathy
- hypertensive cardiac failure or myocardial infarction
- aortic dissection
- pre-eclampsia or eclampsia
- intracerebral haemorrhage with a systolic blood pressure >200 mmHg.

Swallowing assessment should be undertaken with use of a nasal bridle, nasogastric or gastrostomy tube for those unable to feed. Early mobilisation is also advised. In view of an ischaemic stroke, aspirin 300 mg should be given. Adequate blood sugar control is required with a target aim between 4 and 11 mmol/L. Individuals with evidence of acute intracerebral haemorrhage should be referred for neurosurgical intervention.

Transient ischaemic attack

Symptoms
- Speech disturbance, gait disturbance, change in behaviour, altered memory, weakness, numbness

Signs
- Atrial fibrillation, facial weakness, visual field defects, motor weakness

Differentials
- Carotid artery dissection
- Meningitis
- Stroke
- Subarachnoid haemorrhage
- Syncope

How to investigate?
Blood investigations of choice include a full blood count, urea and electrolytes and coagulation profile in addition to lipid studies. Patients with a suspected transient ischaemic attack should undergo ABCD[2] scoring.
- Age >60 years: 1 point
- Blood pressure >140/90 mmHg at initial evaluation: 1 point
- Clinical features of transient ischaemic attack: unilateral weakness (2 points), speech disturbance without weakness (1 point)
- Duration of symptoms: <10 minutes (0 points), 10–59 minutes (1 point), >60 minutes (2 points)
- Diabetes: 1 point

Those with an ABCD[2] score of 4 or more or with crescendo transient ischaemic attacks (namely, two or more in a week) should undergo computed tomography or MRI scanning within at least 24 hours of symptom onset. Those with a lower risk score – namely, an ABCD[2] score of 3 or less – or those presenting more than a week after symptom resolution should undergo investigations ideally within a week. Carotid Doppler ultrasound is an important imaging tool to help determine an individual's need for endarterectomy.

How to manage?

Transient ischaemic attacks should be managed with aspirin 300 mg as soon as possible. Individuals with 70%–99% carotid artery stenosis according to the European Carotid Surgery Trial criteria should undergo carotid endarterectomy within 2 weeks of symptom onset. Those with <70% stenosis should be treated medically with antiplatelet agents, adequate blood pressure control and dietary measures.

Clopidogrel is now recommended as an option to prevent occlusive vascular events:

➲ for people who have had an ischaemic stroke or who have peripheral arterial disease or multivascular disease or

➲ for people who have had a myocardial infarction, only if aspirin is contraindicated or not tolerated.

Modified-release dipyridamole in combination with aspirin is recommended as an option to prevent occlusive vascular events:

➲ for people who have had a transient ischaemic attack or for people who have had an ischaemic stroke only, if clopidogrel is contraindicated or not tolerated.

Modified-release dipyridamole alone is recommended as an option to prevent occlusive vascular events:

➲ for people who have had an ischaemic stroke, only if aspirin and clopidogrel are contraindicated or not tolerated or

➲ for people who have had a transient ischaemic attack, only if aspirin is contraindicated or not tolerated.

Subarachnoid haemorrhage

Symptoms

➲ Headache (thunderclap), dizziness, eye pain, double vision, visual loss, weakness, fits, speech disturbance, nausea, vomiting, neck stiffness

Signs

➲ Hypertension, cranial nerve palsies, papilloedema, hemiparesis

Differentials

➲ Meningitis

➲ Encephalitis

➲ Intracranial haemorrhage

⊃ Ischaemic stroke

⊃ Transient ischaemic attack

How to investigate?

A CT scan of the brain followed by a lumbar puncture, if the scan is negative, are the mainstay investigations. A lumbar puncture should not be performed in cases of elevated intracranial pressure, hydrocephalus or intracranial mass and it helps to determine the presence of red blood cells and xanthochromia. Cerebral angiography should be performed in patients with a subarachnoid haemorrhage to determine the presence and anatomical features of aneurysmal formation. In cases where cerebral angiography cannot be performed, magnetic resonance angiography and computed tomography angiography should be considered.

How to manage?

Monitoring and careful control of blood pressure is important in such cases. Surgical clipping or endovascular coiling should be performed to reduce the risk of re-bleeding. Cerebral vasospasm is a common occurrence after a subarachnoid haemorrhage. This can be appropriately managed through the use of oral nimodipine. Because of the risk of hydrocephalus associated with subarachnoid haemorrhage, temporary or permanent cerebrospinal fluid diversion is required. Seizures should be best controlled with anti-epileptic therapy (see below) and in cases of hyponatraemia, which can occur in up to 30% of cases, patients may benefit from fludrocortisone and hypertonic saline.

Delirium

Symptoms

⊃ Confusion, hallucinations, delusions, sleep disturbance, mood disturbance, speech abnormalities, weakness

Signs

⊃ Fluctuating consciousness level, impaired attention, memory disturbance, altered cognition

Differentials

⊃ Depression

⊃ Psychosis

How to investigate?

Investigations of choice are extensive and include a full blood count, urea and electrolytes, liver and thyroid function tests as well as a CRP. Urine should be screened to exclude infection and drug misuse. Haematinic screening should be performed as well. Imaging via computed tomography or MRI is beneficial in addition to an electroencephalogram. If an underlying cause is unclear, one can consider the use of a lumbar puncture.

How to manage?

Management relies on treatment of the underlying cause. Patients should be reassured through effective communication and reorientation. From a pharmacological perspective, short-term haloperidol or olanzapine can be employed. However, such antipsychotics should be avoided in those with Parkinson's disease or Lewy body dementia.

Status epilepticus

Symptoms
- ➲ Limb jerking, eye twitching, weakness, numbness, visual disturbance, hallucinations (visual or olfactory), lip smacking, speech disturbances

Signs
- ➲ Papilloedema, increased tone, jerk-like movements

Differentials
- ➲ Encephalitis
- ➲ Hypo- or hypernatremia
- ➲ Hypoglycaemia
- ➲ Hypocalcaemia
- ➲ Uraemic encephalopathy
- ➲ Neuroleptic malignant syndrome

How to investigate?

Investigations of choice include a full blood count, urea and electrolytes including serum calcium and magnesium, liver function tests, serum glucose, coagulation profile, anti-convulsant levels and blood and urine toxicology screens. Additional investigations may include a chest X-ray, a CT scan or MRI brain, and lumbar puncture. In cases of refractory status epilepticus, electroencephalogram monitoring is preferred.

How to manage?

It is important to follow the 'ABC' mantra in such cases, ensuring the airway is secured, oxygen administered and intravenous access obtained. Glucose and thiamine should be prescribed if concerns regarding alcohol misuse exist. Regular neurological monitoring is required, with ITU input as necessary.

From a pharmacological perspective, diazepam 10–20 mg per rectum should be administered and repeated 15 minutes later as necessary. Lorazepam 0.1 mg/kg should be started (usually a 4 mg bolus repeated once after 10–20 minutes). Following this, a phenytoin infusion is required, usually at a dose of 15–18 mg/kg and a rate of 50 mg/minute.

Bacterial meningitis

Symptoms

➲ Headache, nausea, fever, rash, photophobia, neck stiffness

Signs

Neck stiffness, cranial nerve palsies, photophobia, non-blanching petechiae, Kernig's sign (painful knee extension when thigh is bent at the hip and the knee is at 90 degrees), Brudziński's sign (involuntary leg lifting when lifting a patient's head when lying supine).

Differentials

➲ Brain abscess
➲ Encephalitis
➲ Brain neoplasm
➲ Subarachnoid haemorrhage

How to investigate?

Investigations of choice include a CT or MRI head, in addition to a lumbar puncture with measurement of cerebrospinal fluid cell count (typically polymorphs), protein (typically elevated), glucose (classically reduced), Gram stain and culture and antigen detection. Blood cultures should also be sent, in addition to a full blood count, urea and electrolytes and C-reactive protein.

How to manage?

Empirical treatment is typically age dependent. Those >1 month but <50 years of age require vancomycin and ceftriaxone or cefotaxime. Those >50 years of age benefit from ampicillin, vancomycin and ceftriaxone or cefotaxime.

In cases of confirmed bacterial meningitis, antibiotics of choice are as follows:

- ◔ Streptococcal – benzylpenicillin/ampicillin or chloramphenicol if penicillin allergic
- ◔ *Haemophilus influenzae* beta lactamase negative – ampicillin or chloramphenicol; beta lactamase positive cases should be treated with ceftriaxone, cefotaxime or meropenem
- ◔ *Escherichia coli* – gentamicin and ceftriaxone or cefotaxime
- ◔ Listeria – gentamicin and benzylpenicillin or ampicillin
- ◔ *Neisseria meningitidis* – benzylpenicllin/ampicillin or ceftriaxone/cefotaxime.

Viral meningitis

Symptoms
- ◔ Nausea, vomiting, neck stiffness, rash, headache, fever

Signs
- ◔ Fever, neck stiffness, confusion, photophobia, seizures, brisk reflexes, rash

Differentials
- ◔ Bacterial meningitis
- ◔ Systemic lupus erythematosus
- ◔ Encephalomyelitis

How to investigate?
Routine blood investigations are essential and include a full blood count, urea and electrolytes and C-reactive protein. Cerebrospinal fluid analysis is key in determining a diagnosis. Cerebrospinal fluid findings include the presence of mononuclear cells with a normal or elevated protein and reduction in glucose. Cerebrospinal fluid should be sent for a polymerase chain reaction test for enteroviruses and herpes virus. Prior to a lumbar puncture, patients should, of course, undergo a CT or MRI head.

How to manage?
Management is virus dependent, with the herpes simplex virus best treated with acyclovir and cases of cytomegalovirus-induced meningitis most appropriately managed with ganciclovir. Patients should also be adequately fluid resuscitated with anti-pyretic therapies and analgesia as needed.

Encephalitis

Symptoms

➲ Fever, headache, nausea, vomiting, muscle aches, personality change, neck pain, photophobia, fits, weakness, skin lesions

Signs

➲ Focal neurological deficit, cranial nerve palsies, dysphagia, skin lesions, ataxia

Differentials

➲ Brain abscess
➲ Hypoglycaemia
➲ Meningitis
➲ Status epilepticus
➲ Subarachnoid haemorrhage
➲ Systemic lupus erythematosus
➲ Toxoplasmosis
➲ Tuberculosis

How to investigate?

Investigations of choice include a CT or MRI head, which will typically demonstrate temporal lobe involvement, in addition to a lumbar puncture if there are no obvious contraindications. Cerebrospinal fluid findings include an elevated protein and a lymphocyte count with a reduction in glucose. Cerebrospinal fluid polymerase chain reaction assay for the herpes simplex virus should of course also be performed. Routine blood investigations should be carried out and these include a full blood count, urea and electrolytes and C-reactive protein.

How to manage?

Treatment is, of course, cause dependent. Management of choice involves intravenous acyclovir in cases of herpes simplex virus–related encephalitis.

Head injury

Symptoms
- Confusion, headache, loss of power or sensation

Signs
- Bleeding, anosmia, hearing loss, pupillary abnormalities, focal neurological deficit, flexor or extensor posturing, tremor, speech disturbance, lucid intervals

Differentials
- Stroke
- Alzheimer's disease
- Acute confusional state
- Epilepsy
- Hydrocephalus
- Subarachnoid haemorrhage
- Subdural haematoma

How to investigate?

Investigations of choice involve a CT head scan and C spine imaging as required. The National Institute for Health and Care Excellence advocates the use of computerised tomography imaging of the head within 1 hour in the following cases:
- Glasgow Coma Scale score <13 when first assessed in the emergency department
- Glasgow Coma Scale score <15 when assessed in the emergency department 2 hours after the injury
- suspected open or depressed skull fracture
- sign of fracture at skull base (haemotympanum, 'panda' eyes, cerebrospinal fluid leakage from ears or nose, Battle's sign)
- post-traumatic seizure
- focal neurological deficit
- one episode of vomiting
- amnesia or loss of consciousness post injury with evidence of coagulopathy.

Of course all patients require blood tests comprising a full blood count, renal profile, liver function tests, coagulation screen and C-reactive protein.

How to manage?

It is important to discuss such patients with neurosurgical specialists and ensure steps are taken towards intubation and ventilation as required.

Raised intracranial pressure

Symptoms
- Headache, drowsiness, vomiting, fits, visual loss

Signs
- Seizures, Cheyne–Stokes respiration, pupillary disturbance, visual field loss, papilloedema

Differentials
- Hydrocephalus
- Stroke
- Meningioma

How to investigate?

Patients should undergo immediate computerised tomography imaging and intracranial pressure monitoring as appropriate. Blood investigations should include a full blood count, urea and electrolytes, coagulation screen and C-reactive protein.

How to manage?

Patients should be appropriately oxygenated and maintained in an euvolaemic state. Seizure activity can exacerbate intracranial pressure and hence anticonvulsants should be instigated. Cerebrospinal fluid can be drained courtesy of the intraventricular catheters used to monitor intracranial pressure. Additional measures include elevation of the head of the bed and analgesia or sedation as required. Medical therapies include the use of diuretics, such as mannitol, which help to decrease the intracranial pressure. Studies have shown that decompressive craniectomies have proven worthwhile in some cases and so consideration of this technique is paramount.

Chapter 5

RHEUMATOLOGY

Septic arthritis

Symptoms

➲ Joint pain, fever, joint swelling, rigors

Signs

➲ Joint swelling, erythema

Differentials

➲ Crystal-induced arthritis
➲ Rheumatoid arthritis
➲ Reactive arthritis
➲ Lyme disease

How to investigate?

Blood investigations of importance include a full blood count, urea and electrolytes, liver function tests, C-reactive protein and erythrocyte sedimentation rate. Blood cultures should also be sent, and synovial fluid aspirated if possible and sent for culture.

How to manage?

Antibiotic treatment relies typically on the use of flucloxacillin or clindamycin if penicillin allergic. It is important to mention that septic joints should be aspirated to dryness.

Chapter 6

ENDOCRINOLOGY

Diabetic ketoacidosis

Symptoms

⮑ Increasing thirst, increasing urinary frequency, weakness, nausea, vomiting, abdominal pain, weight loss, confusion

Signs

⮑ Dehydration, ketotic breath, tachypnoea, hyporeflexia, hypotension, tachycardia, abdominal tenderness

Differentials

⮑ Hyperosmolar hyperglycaemic state
⮑ Acute pancreatitis
⮑ Septic shock
⮑ Urinary tract infection

How to investigate?

Investigations of relevance include a venous and laboratory glucose, in addition to a full blood count, urea and electrolytes, blood cultures, arterial blood gas, ECG, chest X-ray and urine microscopy and culture.

How to manage?

Within the first hour, it is important to commence 0.9% sodium chloride fluid replacement and an insulin infusion of 50 units of actrapid in 50 mL of 0.9% sodium chloride. Patients should undergo regular capillary blood glucose monitoring as well as ketone measurement, in addition to venous bicarbonate, pH and electrolyte monitoring. High-dependency or intensive care input may be required in cases of cardiac or renal co-morbidities, blood ketones >6 mmol/L, a venous bicarbonate below 5 mmol/L, venous pH below 7.1, hypokalaemia, a Glasgow Coma Scale score <12 and hypotension. As insulin drives potassium into cells, potassium replacement is essential and can be instigated as follows:

⮑ potassium 5.5 mmol/L – nil potassium needed
⮑ potassium 3.5–5.5 mmol/L – 40 mmol/L.

As a general rule, fluid replacement should then continue as follows:
⮑ 0.9% sodium chloride 1 L with potassium chloride over next 2 hours
⮑ 0.9% sodium chloride 1 L with potassium chloride over next 2 hours
⮑ 0.9% sodium chloride 1 L with potassium chloride over next 4 hours
⮑ 0.9% sodium chloride 1 L with potassium chloride over next 4 hours
⮑ 0.9% sodium chloride 1 L with potassium chloride over 6 hours.

It is important to note that if blood glucose falls below 14 mmol/L, 10% glucose at a rate of 125 mL/hour should be started.

To ensure adequate thromboprophylaxis, prophylactic low-molecular-weight heparin should be commenced.

Resolution of diabetic ketoacidosis is defined as a ketone level of <0.3 mmol/L and a venous pH >7.3. Once this has occurred and the patient is able to eat and drink, he or she should be transferred to subcutaneous insulin.

Hyperosmolar hyperglycaemic state

Symptoms

- Drowsiness, lethargy, fits, visual disturbance, increasing thirst, increasing urinary frequency, weight loss, weakness

Signs

- Tachycardia, hypotension, dehydration, atypical neurological findings such as upgoing plantars and nystagmus, fever

Differentials

- Diabetes insipidus
- Diabetic ketoacidosis
- Sepsis

How to investigate?

Investigations of choice include a venous blood glucose, urea and electrolytes, serum osmolality measurement, an arterial blood gas, blood ketones and lactate, full blood count, blood cultures, ECG, chest X-ray, urine microscopy and culture and C-reactive protein.

How to manage?

It is important to appreciate the potential severity of a hyperosmolar hyperglycaemic state. High dependency or intensive therapy unit input may be required in case of an osmolality >350 mosmol/kg, serum sodium >160 mmol/L, pH <7.1, hypo- or hyperkalaemia, altered Glasgow Coma Scale score, hypotension, serum creatinine >200 micromol/L and a urine output <0.5 mL/kg/hour. Intravenous 0.9% sodium chloride should be used to restore volume loss as appropriate. Intravenous insulin should only be started if the blood glucose is no longer falling with intravenous fluids alone or if there is significant ketonaemia. Appropriate blood glucose monitoring in addition to regular measurement of urea and electrolytes should occur.

It is important to note that blood glucose should be kept between 10 and 15 mmol/L. Intravenous fluids should be continued until the patient begins eating and drinking.

Thyroid storm or crisis

Symptoms

⮑ Fever, sweating, weight loss, shortness of breath, nausea and vomiting, diarrhoea, abdominal pain, anxiety, fits

Signs

⮑ Hyperpyrexia, haemodynamic instability, atrial flutter or fibrillation, hyperreflexia, seizures, orbital signs in keeping with thyrotoxicosis, goitre

Differentials

⮑ Anxiety
⮑ Hyperthyroidism
⮑ Phaeochromocytoma

How to investigate?

Investigations of choice include thyroid function tests, which typically demonstrate an elevated T3 and T4 level with suppressed thyroid-stimulating hormone levels. Other useful investigations include a full blood count, urea and electrolytes and C-reactive protein. An ECG is essential to help exclude arrhythmias such as atrial fibrillation, which is particularly common.

How to manage?

Because of its clinical severity, high dependency or intensive therapy unit input is strongly recommended. The mainstay form of treatment relies on the use of beta blockers – namely, propranolol, antithyroid drugs, Lugol's iodine or potassium iodide, steroids (which help to decrease the conversion of T4 to T3), aggressive cooling and fluid resuscitation typically with dextrose. The antithyroid drug of choice is propylthiouracil.

Myxoedema crisis

Symptoms
- ➲ Fatigue, cold intolerance, constipation, dry skin, lethargy, weight gain

Signs
- ➲ Hypothermia, hypotension, thickened skin, slow relaxing reflexes, periorbital oedema

Differentials
- ➲ Sick euthyroid syndrome
- ➲ Hypothermia
- ➲ Septic shock

How to investigate?
Patients should undergo measurement of T4, T3 (which are typically low) and thyroid-stimulating hormone measurement (which is classically elevated). Renal function helps to exclude hyponatraemia and acute renal failure in view of reduced perfusion. A full blood count will help to exclude infection and a serum glucose is beneficial in view of the risk of hypoglycaemia. An ECG will often demonstrate bradycardia.

How to manage?
As is the case with thyroid storm/crisis, high dependency or intensive therapy unit input is highly recommended. Fluid resuscitation is paramount and typically involves saline intravenously. Hypothermia should be managed with external warming. Thyroid hormone replacement is of course essential and should be replaced intravenously. Because of the possibility of adrenal insufficiency, steroid replacement may be required.

Addisonian crisis

Symptoms

➲ Nausea, vomiting, abdominal pain

Signs

➲ Abdominal tenderness, haemodynamic instability, hyper- or hypothermia

Differentials

➲ Septic shock

How to investigate?

Investigations of choice include a full blood count to exclude infection as well as serum urea and electrolytes, which will demonstrate hyponatraemia and hyperkalaemia. Serum glucose should be measured, as it is typically reduced. One should determine adrenal insufficiency through measurement of serum cortisol (<20 mcg/dL) and the adrenocorticotropic hormone test. An increase of <9 mcg/dL following adrenocorticotropic hormone administration is diagnostic. In case of infection, blood cultures should be performed.

A CT scan of the abdomen is worthwhile for in-depth visualisation of the adrenal glands and to exclude infiltrative pathology, malignancy or haemorrhage, for example.

How to manage?

Steroid replacement via hydrocortisone or dexamethasone is preferred. Such therapy should be commenced immediately on the basis of clinical suspicion. Aggressive fluid resuscitation is also paramount, with dextrose and saline replacement.

Chapter 7

CARDIOLOGY

Atrial fibrillation

Symptoms

⮞ Palpitations, dyspnoea, dizziness, chest pain, fainting (syncope)

Signs

⮞ Irregularly irregular pulse, tachycardia, signs of heart failure

Differentials

⮞ Atrial flutter
⮞ Atrial tachycardia
⮞ Atrioventricular nodal re-entry tachycardia
⮞ Paroxysmal supraventricular tachycardia
⮞ Wolff–Parkinson–White syndrome

How to investigate?

Of course it goes without saying that an ECG is the gold standard investigation. Blood investigations including a full blood count, urea and electrolytes, troponin, B-type natriuretic peptide level and thyroid function tests are also worthwhile. An echocardiogram will also provide relevant structural details from an imaging perspective.

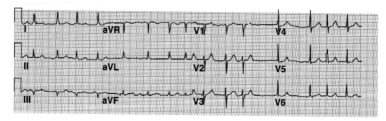

ECG demonstrating evidence of atrial fibrillation

How to manage?

Management relies on rhythm or rate control. Rhythm control is specifically for those who are symptomatic, younger individuals, presenting with lone atrial fibrillation, atrial fibrillation secondary to a treated or corrected precipitant, or with congestive heart failure. Rate control is aimed at those over the age of 65 years, with coronary artery disease, contraindications to anti-arrhythmic drugs and who are unsuitable for cardioversion. Patients should be stratified according to risk of stroke as follows:

⮞ high risk – previous ischaemic stroke or transient ischaemic attack or thromboembolic event, age >75 years with hypertension, diabetes or vascular disease, or clinical evidence of valve disease or heart failure, or impaired left ventricular function on echocardiogram should be anticoagulated with warfarin with a target international normalised ratio of 2–3

➲ moderate risk – age >65 years with no risk factors, age <75 years with hypertension, diabetes or vascular disease should be considered for anticoagulation or aspirin

➲ low risk – age <65 years with no moderate- or high-risk factors should be treated with aspirin 75–300 mg/day if no contraindications.

Pharmacological treatment for rhythm control relies on the use of beta blockers, amiodarone, sotalol or class 1c agents such as flecanide. For rate control, beta blockers, calcium channel blockers, digoxin and amiodarone are worthwhile drugs. Patients who are haemodynamically unstable often require emergency electrical cardioversion.

Atrial flutter

Symptoms
➲ Palpitations, fatigue, dyspnoea, syncope, chest pain, symptoms secondary to hyperthyroidism

Signs
➲ Tachycardia, possible hypotension, bibasal crepitations, signs of hyperthyroidism

Differentials
➲ Atrial fibrillation
➲ Atrial tachycardia

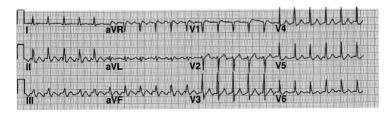

ECG demonstrating evidence of atrial flutter

How to investigate?

An ECG, of course, is the first investigation. Additional investigations include a full blood count, urea and electrolytes, C-reactive protein, thyroid function tests, chest X-ray and echocardiogram.

How to manage?

In cases of haemodynamic compromise, patients should undergo electrical cardioversion. Otherwise, treatment of choice involves beta or calcium channel blockers. As is the case with atrial fibrillation, patients should be anticoagulated in view of stroke prevention.

Third-degree or complete heart block

Symptoms
- ⮕ Fatigue, dizziness, reduced exercise tolerance, chest pain, dyspnoea

Signs
- ⮕ Bradycardia, cannon 'A' waves, tachypnoea, bibasal crepitations, hypotension

Differentials
- ⮕ Myocardial infarction
- ⮕ Myocarditis
- ⮕ Second-degree heart block
- ⮕ Sinus bradycardia

How to investigate?

Investigations of choice include an ECG, full blood count, urea and electrolytes and C-reactive protein. Patients receiving digoxin should undergo digoxin levels and those suspected of myocarditis should be investigated accordingly (*see* later). Additional investigations include a chest X-ray.

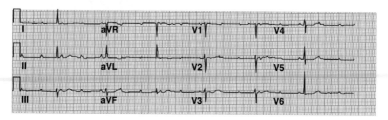

ECG demonstrating complete heart block

How to manage?

Patients should stop offending medications such as digoxin, calcium channel blockers and beta blockers if currently prescribed. Severely symptomatic patients should undergo transcutaneous pacing. Otherwise, the treatment of choice long term is permanent pacemaker insertion.

Acute coronary syndrome

Symptoms
- ⮑ Chest pain or tightness, neck, jaw or arm discomfort, nausea or vomiting, palpitations, dyspnoea, abdominal discomfort

Signs
- ⮑ Pallor, hypo- or hypertension, sweating, pulmonary oedema, cool and clammy skin, existence of third or fourth heart sound

Differentials
- ⮑ Aortic stenosis
- ⮑ Cardiomyopathy
- ⮑ Oesophagitis
- ⮑ Myocarditis
- ⮑ Pericarditis
- ⮑ Cardiac tamponade

How to investigate?

An ECG in addition to a serum troponin level measurement 12 hours from symptom onset. A full blood count helps to exclude anaemia. A chest X-ray and echocardiogram are also worthwhile investigations, in addition to a coronary angiogram or myocardial perfusion scan.

How to manage?

The mainstay form of treatment relies on oxygen, aspirin 300 mg, clopidogrel 300 mg, metoprolol 5–15 mg intravenously or 50–100 mg orally in the absence of bradycardia or hypotension. In the case of ST elevation, presenting within less than 12 hours from symptom onset, individuals should undergo percutaneous coronary intervention and be treated with a glycoprotein IIb/IIIa receptor antagonist intravenously. If percutaneous coronary intervention is not available, patients should be thrombolysed and treated with fondaparinux or low-molecular-weight heparin intravenously. Non-ST elevation should be treated with fondaparinux, or low-molecular-weight heparin. GRACE scoring should be utilised to determine risk of in-hospital death. It comprises the following criteria: age, heart rate, systolic blood pressure, creatinine, Killip class, occurrence of cardiac arrest at admission, ST segment deviation and elevation of cardiac enzymes. Medium- to high-risk individuals should undergo coronary angiography and treatment with a glyco-protein IIb/IIIa receptor antagonist intravenously.

Additional treatments in all of the cases mentioned here include a statin and an angiotensin-converting enzyme inhibitor.

Tachycardia

Symptoms
- ➲ Dyspnoea, light-headedness, dizziness, chest tightness

Signs
- ➲ Rapid pulse rate, hypotension

Differentials
- ➲ Atrial fibrillation
- ➲ Atrial flutter
- ➲ Atrial tachycardia
- ➲ Congestive heart failure
- ➲ Myocardial infarction
- ➲ Supraventricular tachycardia
- ➲ Ventricular tachycardia
- ➲ Ventricular fibrillation

How to investigate?
Investigations of choice include a full blood count, urea and electrolytes and thyroid function tests, in addition to an ECG, of course.

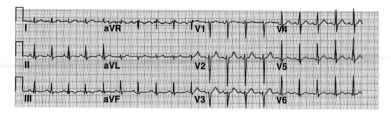

ECG demonstrating sinus tachycardia

How to manage?

Management as per the UK Resuscitation Council is as follows.

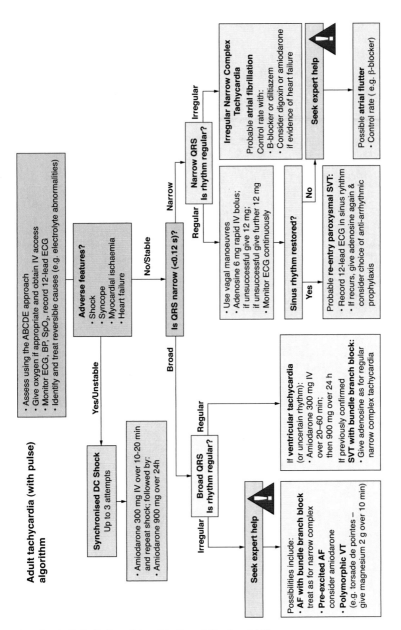

Reproduced with the kind permission of the Resuscitation Council (UK)

Bradycardia

Symptoms

➲ Faints, dizziness, light-headedness, chest pain, shortness of breath

Signs

➲ Slow heart rate, pulmonary oedema, dyspnoea

Differentials

➲ Hypoglycaemia
➲ Hypothermia
➲ Hypothyroidism
➲ Myxoedema coma

How to investigate?

Investigations of choice include a full blood count, urea and electrolytes including calcium and magnesium, serum glucose and thyroid function tests, in addition to an ECG.

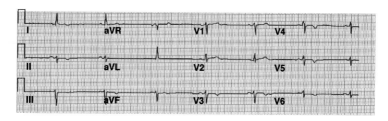

ECG demonstrating evidence of bradycardia

How to manage?

Management as per the UK Resuscitation Council is as follows.

Adult bradycardia algorithm

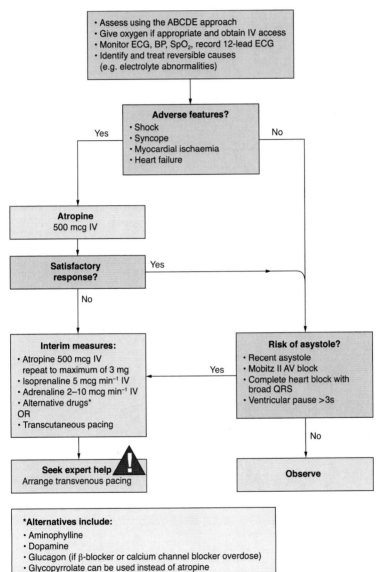

Reproduced with the kind permission of the Resuscitation Council (UK)

Cardiac arrest

How to investigate?

Investigations of choice include a full blood count, urea and electrolytes including calcium and magnesium, cardiac enzymes, thyroid function tests, toxicology screen and arterial blood gas. Imaging of choice includes a chest X-ray and an echocardiogram.

How to manage?

In accordance with the UK Resuscitation Council, the following algorithm helps to highlight the management of ventricular fibrillation or ventricular tachycardia and pulseless electrical activity or asystole.

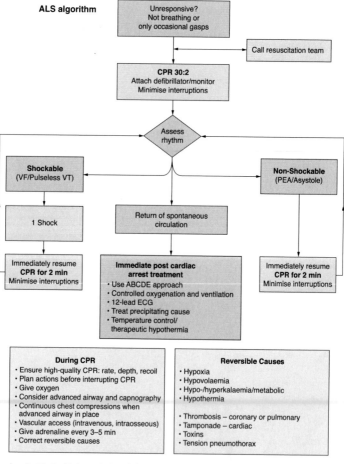

Reproduced with the kind permission of the Resuscitation Council (UK)

Heart failure

Symptoms
- ➲ Dyspnoea, orthopnoea, chest pain, chest tightness, palpitations, nausea, vomiting, fatigue

Signs
- ➲ Elevated venous pressure, cyanosis, diminished pulse volume, ascites, wheeze, crepitations, oedema, hepatomegaly, third heart sound, loud P_2 (pulmonary component of the second heart sound), mitral or tricuspid regurgitation

Differentials
- ➲ Acute respiratory distress syndrome
- ➲ Chronic obstructive pulmonary disease
- ➲ Myocardial infarction
- ➲ Pneumonia
- ➲ Pulmonary oedema
- ➲ Respiratory failure

How to investigate?
Investigations of choice include a full blood count, urea and electrolytes, liver function tests and B-type natriuretic peptide level. In addition, patients require an ECG, echocardiogram and chest X-ray. An arterial blood gas allows for determination of degree of oxygenation and acid base status.

How to manage?
Patients should be adequately oxygenated, with saturations maintained between 95% and 98%. Ventilatory support may be indicated, which is best achieved through continuous positive airway pressure. This method reduces the need for endotracheal intubation and mechanical ventilation. Patients are often restless and require morphine to assist their breathing compromise. Vasodilator therapy is often needed in patients with acute heart failure and typically involves a glyceryl trinitrate infusion, being mindful of blood pressure. In the acute phase, angiotensin-converting enzyme inhibitors are generally not indicated but often have a role to play in chronic presentations. Diuretic therapy is a must and is chosen according to presentation severity.
- ➲ Moderate: typically furosemide orally or intravenously
- ➲ Severe: furosemide infusion or bumetanide
- ➲ Refractory cases: typically metalozone or spironolactone; liaise with high

dependency or intensive therapy unit for consideration of dopamine, dobutamine or ultrafiltration.

Beta blocker therapy is only ever indicated in cases of chronic heart failure.

Those with refractory acute heart failure or end-stage heart failure can benefit from intra-aortic balloon counterpulsation or ventricular assist devices.

Surgical intervention may be employed in cases of acute heart failure secondary to:

➲ multi-vessel disease
➲ ventricular septal defects
➲ acute valvular failure or thrombosis
➲ aneurysmal rupture.

Heart transplantation is considered in cases of severe acute heart failure with a poor outcome.

Hypertensive crisis

Symptoms

➲ Chest pain, headaches, visual disturbance, limb weakness, sweating, palpitations

Signs

➲ Eye signs: silver wiring, arteriovenous nipping, microaneurysm formation, haemorrhage, cotton wool spots, exudates, papilloedema
➲ Diminished or delayed femoral pulses, carotid bruits, renal artery bruit, fourth heart sound, displaced apex

Differentials

➲ Cardiomyopathy
➲ Heart failure
➲ Hyperthyroidism
➲ Myocardial infarction
➲ Stroke

How to investigate?

Investigations of choice include a full blood count, urea and electrolytes, urinalysis and an ECG. Patients with neurological symptoms or signs should undergo a CT head scan. A chest X-ray or chest CT scan should be requested in cases of suspected aortic dissection.

How to manage?
It is generally regarded that anti-hypertensive therapy should be reserved for patients with a diastolic greater than 120 mmHg, with an aim to reduce pressure by 10%–15% in the first 24 hours. Agents of choice typically include nitroprusside or labetalol.

Infective endocarditis

Symptoms
- ⊃ Fever, weight loss, shortness of breath, headache, joint pain, muscle ache, cough, sweats, chest pain

Signs
- ⊃ Petechial rash, splinter haemorrhages, Osler's nodes, Janeway lesions, Roth's spots, focal neurological deficits secondary to emboli, signs of heart failure, finger clubbing, splenomegaly, fever

Differentials
- ⊃ Atrial myxoma
- ⊃ Lyme disease
- ⊃ Reactive arthritis
- ⊃ Systemic lupus erythematosus

How to investigate?
An echocardiogram, initially transthoracic should be performed as soon as possible. If initially negative then this should be repeated or a transoesophageal echocardiogram should be requested. Blood investigations include a full blood count, urea and electrolytes, C-reactive protein and blood cultures, which should be taken from peripheral sites ideally aseptically before treatment has been started. Those with negative blood cultures should undergo serology for Coxiella and Bartonella. Urine should be screened for protein and blood. A chest X-ray can help to exclude embolic phenomenon such as abscesses.

How to manage?
While awaiting blood culture results, patients in the acute setting should be treated as follows.

➲ Native valve endocarditis:
- indolent presentation – amoxicillin and gentamicin
- severe sepsis – vancomycin and gentamicin
- severe sepsis and risk factors for Enterobacteriaceae and Pseudomonas – vancomycin and meropenem
- prosthetic valve endocarditis or negative blood cultures – vancomycin, gentamicin and rifampicin.

Acute myocarditis

Symptoms
➲ Chest pain, fever, sweats, dyspnoea, 'flu-like' symptoms

Signs
➲ Tachycardia, mitral regurgitation, lymphadenopathy, rash

Differentials
➲ Cardiac tamponade
➲ Cardiogenic shock
➲ Cardiomyopathy

How to investigate?
Investigations of choice include a serum troponin and creatine kinase. Other useful investigations include a full blood count, C-reactive protein and erythrocyte sedimentation rate, as well as viral antibodies such as Coxsackie, cytomegalovirus, Epstein–Barr, hepatitis and influenza. An ECG will demonstrate possible tachycardia, non-specific ST-T wave changes and in some cases bundle branch block. An echocardiogram helps to determine the left ventricular ejection fraction and hence subsequent treatment. In addition, a cardiac MRI is a very sensitive test for detecting acute myocarditis. In reality, the gold standard investigation is an endomyocardial biopsy but it is poorly sensitive and poorly specific.

How to manage?
In those with an ejection fraction less than 40%, treatment of choice comprises angiotensin-converting enzyme inhibitors plus beta blocker therapy, in addition to diuretics. Immunosuppressive therapy is not warranted.

Acute pericarditis

Symptoms
- Palpitations, chest pain classically worse on inspiration, fever, dyspnoea, anxiety, confusion

Signs
- Pericardial rub, tachycardia, fever

Differentials
- Angina
- Aortic dissection
- Aortic stenosis
- Oesophageal rupture
- Gastritis
- Gastro-oesophageal reflux disease
- Myocardial infarction
- Peptic ulcer disease
- Pulmonary embolism

How to investigate?
An ECG should be performed in addition to an echocardiogram. Blood investigations should be performed, including an erythrocyte sedimentation rate, C-reactive protein, lactate dehydrogenase, full blood count, urea and electrolytes and serum troponin. A chest X-ray in addition to a CT scan plus or minus an MRI to exclude an effusion should be requested.

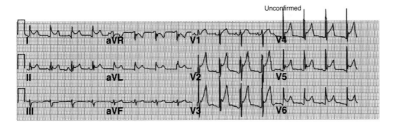

ECG demonstrating evidence of acute pericarditis

How to manage?
Non-steroidal anti-inflammatory drugs are the mainstay form of treatment. As an alternative, colchicine is a useful agent.

Cardiac tamponade

Symptoms

⊃ Dyspnoea, weight loss, fatigue, chest pain, night sweats, fever

Signs

⊃ Tachycardia, hepatomegaly, diminished heart sounds, hypotension, elevated jugular venous pressure, pulsus paradoxus

Differentials

⊃ Cardiogenic shock
⊃ Pericarditis
⊃ Pulmonary embolism
⊃ Tension pneumothorax

How to investigate?

Investigations of choice include an ECG, chest X-ray and echocardiogram, with consideration of a CT scan plus or minus an MRI. Blood investigations involve a full blood count, urea and electrolytes and C-reactive protein.

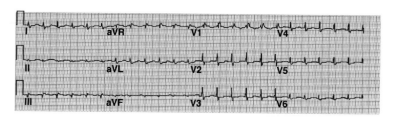

ECG demonstrating evidence of cardiac tamponade

How to manage?

Management relies on pericardiocentesis.

Pericardial effusion

Symptoms

⊃ Chest pain, light-headedness, palpitations, cough, dyspnoea

Signs

⊃ Hypotension, muffled heart sounds, elevated jugular venous pressure, pulsus paradoxus, pericardial rub, tachycardia

Differentials
- ⊃ Cardiac tamponade
- ⊃ Cardiomyopathy
- ⊃ Myocardial infarction
- ⊃ Pericarditis
- ⊃ Pulmonary oedema
- ⊃ Pulmonary embolism

How to investigate?
Blood investigations of choice include a full blood count, renal profile, erythrocyte sedimentation rate, C-reactive protein and autoimmune profile. Cardiac enzyme studies are also worthwhile. Pericardial fluid analysis is important and involves measurement of lactate dehydrogenase, cell count, Gram stain, culture and cytology. Imaging of choice includes a chest X-ray, ECG, echocardiogram and CT scan or MRI. The latter is particularly useful in cases of loculated effusions.

How to manage?
Medical therapy relies upon the use of non-steroidal anti-inflammatory drugs, colchicine or steroids. Antibiotic usage is often reserved for purulent or tuberculous cases. Non-medical intervention is typically in the form of pericardiocentesis, pericardiotomy and pericardiostomy or video-assisted thoracic surgery. Classically effusions are drained when >20 mm on echocardiography.

Cardiogenic shock

Symptoms
- ⊃ Chest pain, neck pain, nausea or vomiting, sweating, syncope, palpitations

Signs
- ⊃ Cyanosis, cool peripheries, hypotension, tachycardia, diminished peripheral pulses, crepitations, elevated jugular venous pressure, third and fourth heart sound, low urine output

Differentials
- ⊃ Myocardial infarction
- ⊃ Pulmonary oedema
- ⊃ Pulmonary embolism
- ⊃ Septic shock

How to investigate?

Blood investigations should include a full blood count, urea and electrolytes, liver function tests, coagulation screen and cardiac enzyme markers. Measurement of serum lactate and B-type natriuretic peptide is also beneficial. Additionally, patients should undergo an ECG, echocardiogram, chest X-ray, and coronary angiography in cases of cardiogenic shock post-myocardial ischaemia or infarction. Haemodynamic assessment is maintained through the use of pulmonary artery catheterisation.

How to manage?

In cases of cardiogenic shock secondary to a myocardial infarction, patients should be treated with aspirin, clopidogrel and heparin. In addition, insulin therapy has been shown to enhance survival in hyperglycaemic myocardial infarction patients. Patients also require inotropic and vasopressor support. Agents of choice include noradrenaline, dopamine and dobutamine. Mechanical support for cardiogenic shock relies upon the use of intra-aortic balloon counterpulsation.

Chapter 8

HAEMATOLOGY

Sickle-cell disease

Symptoms
➔ Pain in any body part, fever, shortness of breath, limb weakness, visual loss, priapism in males, haematuria, cough, haemoptysis

Signs
➔ Scleral icterus, haemodynamic instability, fever, signs of heart failure, signs of pneumonia, splenomegaly, focal neurological deficits, joint deformities

Differentials
➔ Haemolytic anaemia
➔ Leukaemia
➔ Osteomyelitis
➔ Pulmonary embolism
➔ Septic arthritis

How to investigate?
Investigations of choice include a chest X-ray, arterial blood gas, liver function tests, serum amylase, full blood count including reticulocyte count and blood film, blood and urine cultures, parvovirus B19 serology and abdominal ultrasound. In the case of neurological symptoms, a CT or MRI brain is advised.

How to manage?
Oxygen and analgesia is the mainstay form of treatment in such cases. It is important to adequately monitor pain, respiratory rate and sedation every 20 minutes until well controlled. Pain relief is typically governed by the World Health Organization's analgesic ladder, which involves the following steps.
➔ Step 1: mild pain – non-opioid plus or minus adjuvant
➔ Step 2: moderate pain – weak opioid (or low dose of strong opioid) plus or minus non-opioid plus or minus adjuvant
➔ Step 3: severe pain – strong opioid plus or minus non-opioid plus or minus adjuvant

Management of a sickle-cell crisis is governed as follows.
➔ Rapid clinical assessment.
➔ If pain severe and oral analgesia not effective, give strong opioids:
  ● morphine 0.1 mg/kg intravenously or subcutaneously, repeated every 20 minutes until pain controlled; then 0.05–0.1 mg/kg every 2–4 hours intravenously, subcutaneously or orally – consider patient-controlled analgesia, or

- diamorphine 0.1 mg/kg intravenously or subcutaneously repeated every 20 minutes until pain controlled; then 0.05–0.1 mg/kg every 2–4 hours intravenously or subcutaneously – consider patient-controlled analgesia.
➲ Give adjuvant non-opioid analgesia: paracetamol, ibuprofen, diclofenac.
➲ Prescribe laxatives routinely and other adjuvants as necessary:
  - laxatives: lactulose 10 mL twice a day, senna 2–4 tablets once daily, docusate 100 mg twice a day
  - antipruritics: hydroxyzine 25 mg twice a day
  - anti-emetics: prochlorperazine 5–10 mg three times daily, cyclizine 50 mg three times daily
  - anxiolytics: haloperidol 1–3 mg orally or intramuscularly twice a day.
➲ Monitor pain, sedation, vital signs, respiratory rate and oxygen saturations every 30 minutes until pain controlled and stable, and then every 2 hours.
➲ Give rescue doses of analgesia every 30 minutes for breakthrough pains: 50% of maintenance dose.
➲ If respiratory rate less than 10 breaths per minute, omit maintenance analgesia. If severe respiratory depression or sedation, give naloxone 100 mcg intravenously, repeating every 2 minutes as necessary.
➲ Consider reducing analgesia after 2–3 days and replacing injections with equivalent dose of oral opiate.
➲ Discharge patient when pain controlled and improving without analgesia or on acceptable doses of oral analgesia.

Additional management relies on the use of intravenous fluids in cases where the patient is unable to drink, and broad-spectrum antibiotics if the patient is febrile (temperature greater than 38°C) with potential chest symptoms. Blood transfusion should be used as a treatment for symptomatic anaemia and should be leucodepleted and matched for Rh and Kell antigens.

Neutropenic sepsis

Symptoms

➲ Fever, fatigue, weakness, skin abscesses or rash, cough, dyspnoea, swallowing disturbance

Signs

➲ Skin rash or abscess, fever, ulcers, lymphadenopathy, splenomegaly

Differentials

➲ Acute lymphocytic leukaemia
➲ Acute myeloid leukaemia
➲ Aplastic anaemia
➲ HIV
➲ Lymphoma
➲ Systemic lupus erythematosus
➲ Hodgkin's disease

How to investigate?

Investigations of choice include a full blood count, urea and electrolytes, liver function tests, C-reactive protein, serum lactate and blood cultures. Patients will also benefit from a chest X-ray.

How to manage?

Antibiotics are the mainstay form of treatment, with the use of piperacillin and tazobactam.

It is important to note how to recognise and manage sepsis as a general rule. Sepsis is regarded as a temperature >38°C, hypothermia, tachycardia, hypotension (typically a systolic blood pressure of <90 mmHg and mean arterial pressure of <70 mmHg), tachypnoea, confusion, significant oedema and hyperglycaemia. Blood investigations characteristically demonstrate a leukocytosis or leukopenia with a raised C-reactive protein and procalcitonin. Additional diagnostic criteria involve hypoxia, oliguria, a creatinine increase >0.5 mg/dL, disturbed coagulation (international normalised ratio >1.5), ileus, thrombocytopenia and hyperbilirubinaemia. There may also be hyperlactataemia with decreased capillary refill.

The management of sepsis relies on adequate resuscitation in those with hypotension or an elevated serum lactate >4 mmol/L, aiming for a central venous pressure of 8–12 mmHg, mean arterial pressure of 65 mmHg, urine output >0.5 mL/kg/hour and central venous oxygen saturation of >70%. If such venous saturation is not achieved then one should consider further fluid, with transfusion of packed red blood cells plus or minus a dobutamine infusion. Antibiotic usage should be started early, ensuring blood cultures are taken beforehand.

In order to aim for a mean arterial pressure of >65 mmHg, vasopressors of choice include norepinephrine and dopamine. Dobutamine should be used as inotropic support in patients with myocardial dysfunction. In cases where hypotension responds poorly to adequate fluid resuscitation and vasopressors, intravenous hydrocortisone should be used. Red blood cells should be given in cases of a haemoglobin decrease to <7 g/dL. Platelets are transfused when counts are typically less than 30×10^9/L. Intravenous insulin should be commenced to control hyperglycaemia. Intermittent haemodialysis or continuous veno-venous hemofiltration should be considered as a form of renal replacement. Deep vein thrombosis prophylaxis should be initiated in addition to stress ulcer prophylaxis.

Haemolytic anaemia

Symptoms
- ⮑ Dyspnoea, chest pain, weakness, fatigue, abdominal pain, dark urine, leg ulcers

Signs
- ⮑ Pallor, tachycardia, tachypnoea, hypotension, jaundice, splenomegaly, leg ulceration, abdominal tenderness

Differentials
- ⮑ Disseminated intravascular coagulation
- ⮑ Systemic lupus erythematosus
- ⮑ Thrombotic thrombocytopenic purpura

How to investigate?
Investigations of choice include a full blood count, blood film, lactate dehydrogenase, serum haptoglobins (typically reduced) and serum bilirubin (elevated). Additional investigations include a direct antiglobulin test, cold agglutin and sickle-cell screen, as well as a glucose-6-phosphate dehydrogenase screen.

How to manage?
Management relies on the use of steroids in cases of autoimmune haemolytic anaemia. Folic acid is often prescribed because of folate consumption during haemolysis. Intravenous immune globulin is worthwhile in some cases but results

are not always so promising. Blood transfusions should generally be avoided unless patients are experiencing angina or are cardiovascularly compromised.

Thrombocytopenia

Symptoms
- ⊃ Bleeding, bruising, joint discomfort

Signs
- ⊃ Petechiae, purpura, gingival bleeding, retinal haemorrhage, neurological deficit, splenomegaly

Differentials
- ⊃ Immune thrombocytopenic purpura
- ⊃ Thrombotic thrombocytopenic purpura
- ⊃ Haemolytic uraemic syndrome
- ⊃ Von Willebrand's disease

How to investigate?
Investigations of choice include a full blood count, blood film and bleeding time measurement, in addition to urea and electrolytes, C-reactive protein and coagulation profile.

How to manage?
Management is dependent on the cause. Beneficial treatments include steroids, in addition to other immunosuppressive therapy such as azathioprine, cyclophosphamide and rituximab. Intravenous immune globulin therapy may also prove promising. Failing this, patients should undergo a splenectomy. Patients also show particular benefit from plasma exchange–based intervention. In the case of Von Willebrand's disease, patients benefit from the use of desmopressin (DDAVP).

Hyperviscosity syndrome

Symptoms
- ➲ Bleeding, visual loss, weakness, headaches, fits

Signs
- ➲ Bruising, epistaxis, limb weakness, ataxia, nystagmus

Differentials
- ➲ Congestive cardiac failure
- ➲ Pulmonary oedema
- ➲ Stroke

How to investigate?

Blood investigations should include a full blood count, renal profile, coagulation screen and serum viscosity, in addition to a blood film. In cases of new-onset confusion, patients should undergo a CT head scan. A chest X-ray may demonstrate evidence of infection or pulmonary oedema.

How to manage?

The treatment of choice is plasmapheresis.

Tumour lysis syndrome

Symptoms
- ➲ Abdominal pain, urinary symptoms, weakness, lethargy, nausea or vomiting, muscle cramps, fits

Signs
- ➲ Tetany, seizures, skin lesions, dyspnoea, pulmonary oedema, hypertension

Differentials
- ➲ Acute renal failure

How to investigate?

Blood investigations of choice include a full blood count, renal profile including phosphate, calcium and uric acid, in addition to a serum lactate dehydrogenase. Patients should also undergo cardiac monitoring in view of electrolyte disturbances, in addition to urine pH monitoring.

How to manage?

Patients with tumour lysis syndrome should undergo urgent fluid resuscitation, in view of associated renal dysfunction. In addition, allopurinol should be instigated to aid in reducing urate levels.

Disseminated intravascular coagulation

Symptoms

Symptoms are typical of the underlying condition. In the acute phase there may be bleeding and petechiae. Dyspnoea, cough, haemoptysis may also be common symptoms, in addition to confusion and weakness

Signs

⮕ Focal neurological deficits, hypotension, tachycardia, signs of acute respiratory distress syndrome, haematemesis, petechiae, jaundice, cyanosis, skin necrosis

Differentials

⮕ Haemolytic uraemic syndrome
⮕ Idiopathic thrombocytopenic purpura
⮕ Thrombotic thrombocytopenic purpura
⮕ Heparin-induced thrombocytopenia

How to investigate?

Investigations of choice include a full blood count, platelet count, D-dimer, prothrombin time, fibrinogen level, urea and electrolytes and C-reactive protein. A scoring system based on these variables exists and involves the following.

⮕ Risk assessment: does the patient have an underlying disorder known to be associated with overt disseminated intravascular coagulation (DIC)?
  ● If yes: proceed
  ● If no: do not use this algorithm.
⮕ Order global coagulation tests (prothrombin time, platelet count, fibrinogen, fibrin-related marker)
⮕ Score the test results:
  ● platelet count ($>100 \times 10^9/L$ = 0, $<100 \times 10^9/L$ = 1, $<50 \times 10^9/L$ = 2)
  ● elevated fibrin marker (e.g. D-dimer, fibrin degradation products) (no increase = 0, moderate increase = 2, strong increase = 3)
  ● prolonged prothrombin time (<3 seconds = 0, >3 but <6 seconds = 1, >6 seconds = 2)
  ● fibrinogen level ($>1\,g/L$ = 0, $<1\,g/L$ = 1).

- ⊃ Calculate score:
  - >5 compatible with overt DIC: repeat score daily
  - <5 suggestive for non-overt DIC: repeat next 1–2 days.

How to manage?

Treatment relies on management of the underlying condition. Platelet transfusion should be instigated in those with DIC and bleeding as well as a platelet count of less than 50×10^9/L. In bleeding patients with DIC, a prolonged prothrombin time and activated partial thromboplastin time, fresh frozen plasma should be administered. If administration of fresh frozen plasma is not possible, prothrombin complex concentrate is a suitable alternative. Severe hypofibrinogenaemia that persists despite fresh frozen plasma replacement can be treated with fibrinogen concentrate or cryoprecipitate.

In situations where thrombosis is a major concern, heparin as a therapeutic dose should be administered.

Patients severely septic with DIC should be treated with recombinant human activated protein C. This treatment is contraindicated in those patients at high risk of bleeding and with a platelet count of less than 30×10^9/L.

Malaria

Symptoms

- ⊃ Cough, fatigue, chills, joint and muscle pain, fever, sweats, headache, nausea, vomiting, jaundice, diarrhoea

Signs

- ⊃ Seizures, signs of renal failure and pulmonary oedema, hepatosplenomegaly

Differentials

- ⊃ Dengue fever
- ⊃ Infective endocarditis
- ⊃ Typhoid fever
- ⊃ Leptospirosis

How to investigate?

Investigations of choice include a full blood count (anaemia and thrombocytopenia typically seen), reticulocyte count (in view of haemolysis) urea and electrolytes, liver function tests, serum glucose, an arterial blood gas, C-reactive protein and lactate dehydrogenase. Blood cultures should be obtained in addition of course to thick and thin blood smears. Depending on symptomatology, a chest X-ray and a CT head scan should be considered.

How to manage?

Management relies upon appropriate patient assessment with utilisation of the 'ABC' approach. Depending on species, treatment is as follows.

➡ *Plasmodium falciparum* – chloroquine or hydroxychloroquine
  - In those who are chloroquine resistant, treatment involves artemisinin combination therapies or atovaquone–proguanil. Other options include quinine plus doxycycline or tetracycline.
  - In severe disease, patients should undergo intravenous treatment typically with artesunate or quinine and doxycycline until the parasite count is <1% and the patient is able to tolerate oral therapy.
➡ *Plasmodium ovale* – chloroquine plus primaquine
➡ *Plasmodium vivax* – chloroquine plus primaquine
➡ *Plasmodium malariae* – chloroquine

Chapter 9

ADDITIONAL MEDICAL EMERGENCIES

Hypovolaemic shock

Symptoms

- ⇒ Weakness, light-headedness, symptoms of underlying cause (e.g. haematemesis or melaena in cases of a gastrointestinal bleed)

Signs

- ⇒ Tachycardia, hypotension, cool and clammy skin, delayed capillary refill, oliguria, altered mental status

Differentials

- ⇒ Abdominal aneurysm
- ⇒ Peptic ulcer disease

How to investigate?

Investigations of choice include a full blood count, urea and electrolytes, serum glucose, coagulation profile, an arterial blood gas, urinalysis and, if female, a pregnancy test to exclude an ectopic pregnancy.

Depending on cause, additional investigations may include an abdominal ultrasound (to exclude an abdominal aortic aneurysm), or an endoscopy in those suspected of a gastrointestinal bleed.

How to manage?

Patients should be assessed courtesy of the 'ABC' approach. Rapid fluid resuscitation is essential, either crystalloid or colloid based, and typically 500 mL in the first instance. It is important to note that treatment of the underlying cause is essential in such cases and that over-rapid correction may lead to pulmonary oedema. For hypotension refractory to volume resuscitation, vasopressors should be started, such as noradrenaline or dopamine.

Septic shock

Please refer to the section 'Neutropenic sepsis' (*see* p. 74).

Anaphylaxis

Symptoms

➲ Urticaria, itch, swelling, throat tightness, dyspnoea, chest pain, flushing, headache, dizziness, nausea and vomiting, abdominal pain

Signs

➲ Angioedema, wheeze, stridor, tachycardia, hypotension, urticaria, erythema

Differentials

➲ Phaeochromocytoma
➲ Angioedema

How to investigate?

Investigations include a full blood count, urea and electrolytes, ECG, chest X-ray and arterial blood gas. Mast cell tryptase is a useful investigation of choice to help confirm the diagnosis.

How to manage?

Management as per the UK Resuscitation Council is as follows.

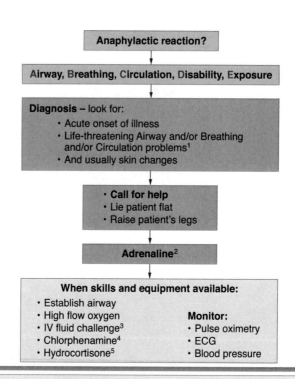

Anaphylactic reaction?

Airway, Breathing, Circulation, Disability, Exposure

Diagnosis – look for:
- Acute onset of illness
- Life-threatening Airway and/or Breathing and/or Circulation problems[1]
- And usually skin changes

- **Call for help**
- Lie patient flat
- Raise patient's legs

Adrenaline[2]

When skills and equipment available:
- Establish airway
- High flow oxygen
- IV fluid challenge[3]
- Chlorphenamine[4]
- Hydrocortisone[5]

Monitor:
- Pulse oximetry
- ECG
- Blood pressure

---

[1] **Life-threatening problems:**
Airway: swelling, hoarseness, stridor
Breathing: rapid breathing, wheeze, fatigue, cyanosis, SpO_2 <92%, confusion
Circulation: pale, clammy, low blood pressure, faintness, drowsy/coma

[2] **Adrenaline** *(give IM unless experienced with IV adrenaline)*
IM doses of 1:1000 adrenaline (repeat after 5 min if no better)
- Adult: 500 micrograms IM (0.5 mL)
- Child more than 12 years: 500 micrograms IM (0.5 mL)
- Child 6–12 years: 300 micrograms IM (0.3 mL)
- Child less than 6 years: 150 micrograms IM (0.15 mL)

Adrenaline IV to be given **only by experienced specialists**
Titrate: Adults 50 micrograms; Children 1 microgram/kg

[3] **IV fluid challenge:**
Adult–500–1000 mL
Child–crystalloid 20 mL/kg

Stop IV colloid
if this might be the cause
of anaphylaxis

	[4] Chlorphenamine (IM or slow IV)	[5] Hydrocortisone (IM or slow IV)
Adult or child more than 12 years:	10 mg	200 mg
Child 6–12 years:	5 mg	100 mg
Child 6 months to 6 years:	2.5 mg	50 mg
Child less than 6 months:	250 micrograms/kg	25 mg

Reproduced with the kind permission of the Resuscitation Council (UK)

Aspirin overdose

Symptoms
- Tinnitus, fever, sweating, visual disturbance, fits, nausea, vomiting, abdominal pain

Signs
- Hyperventilation, dyspnoea, fever, haemodynamic instability, arrhythmias, tremor, neurological deficit, seizures, abdominal tenderness, dehydration

Differentials
- Alcohol misuse
- Diabetic ketoacidosis
- Acute respiratory distress syndrome

How to investigate?
Investigations of choice include a full blood count, urea and electrolytes, liver function tests, coagulation screen, serum glucose and C-reactive protein in addition, of course, to regular salicylate-level monitoring. An arterial blood gas is key to help confirm or exclude the presence of a respiratory alkalosis, which occurs initially and is followed by a metabolic acidosis.

How to manage?
Management is salicylate-level dependent.
- Mild poisoning: salicylate level 300–600 mg/L, requires rehydration with oral or intravenous fluids
- Moderate poisoning: salicylate level 600–800 mg/L, relies on the use of urinary alkalinisation with sodium bicarbonate
- Severe poisoning: salicylate level >800 mg/L, focuses on the use of haemodialysis in addition to sodium bicarbonate

Paracetamol overdose

Symptoms
➲ Nausea, vomiting, loss of appetite, sweating, abdominal pain, jaundice

Signs
➲ Abdominal tenderness (typically right upper quadrant), jaundice, haemodynamic instability

Differentials
➲ Acute tubular necrosis
➲ Pancreatitis
➲ Peptic ulcer disease
➲ Viral hepatitis

How to investigate?
Investigations of choice include a full blood count, urea and electrolytes, liver function tests, coagulation screen and paracetamol level in addition to a serum glucose and arterial blood gas to exclude the existence of a metabolic acidosis.

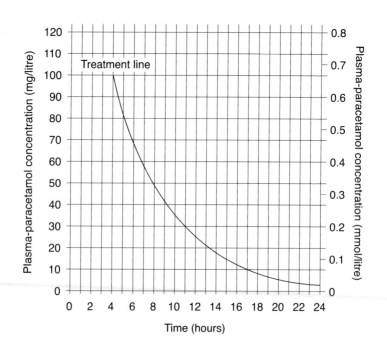

How to manage?

In accordance with the Medicines and Healthcare Products Regulatory Agency, patients should be managed with acetylcysteine irrespective of the plasma paracetamol level in circumstances where the overdose is staggered or there is doubt over the time of paracetamol ingestion; or a paracetamol overdose with a timed plasma paracetamol concentration on or above a single treatment line joining points of 100 mg/L at 4 hours and 15 mg/L at 15 hours of the nomogram regardless of risk factors of hepatotoxicity.

It is now recommended that the administration of the first dose of intravenous acetylcysteine should last 1 hour in duration.

Opioid overdose

Symptoms
➲ Confusion, reduced bowel movement, fits

Signs
➲ Miosis, dysrhythmias, reduced respiratory rate, needle track marks

Differentials
➲ Alcohol misuse
➲ Diabetic ketoacidosis
➲ Electrolyte disturbances such as hypoglycaemia
➲ Hypothermia
➲ Stroke
➲ Other drug toxicity such as barbiturates or benzodiazepines

How to investigate?
Blood investigations involve a full blood count, urea and electrolytes, liver function tests, C-reactive protein and arterial blood gas. A urine drug screen is certainly worthwhile.

How to manage?
Appropriate patient assessment using the 'ABC' approach, in addition to naloxone 0.4–2 mg intravenously, intramuscularly or subcutaneously every 2–3 minutes up to a maximum of 10 mg. Consideration of an infusion should be given to patients exposed to long-acting opioids.

Hypothermia

Symptoms
- ➲ Confusion, dizziness, dyspnoea, mood disturbance, speech disturbance

Signs
- ➲ Temperature below 35°C, dysarthria, tachypnoea, ataxia, hyporeflexia, arrhythmias, oliguria, hypotension, fixed pupils

Differentials
- ➲ Stroke
- ➲ Alcohol toxicity
- ➲ Drug toxicity (e.g. barbiturates, benzodiazepines)

How to investigate?
Ideally, patients should undergo core temperature measurement, although this is not always possible in addition to cardiac monitoring. (Take note of cardiac dysrhythmias and treat accordingly!) Patients require blood investigations – namely, a full blood count, urea and electrolytes, coagulation screen, C-reactive protein and serum glucose. A chest X-ray and CT head scan may also be worthwhile.

How to manage?
Treatment of the underlying cause is key in such situations and patients should undergo active external and minimally invasive rewarming. Intravenous fluids should be warmed to a temperature of 38°C–42°C to prevent further heat loss. Extracorporeal membrane oxygenation or cardiopulmonary bypass should be considered for patients with hypothermia and cardiac instability. Research has shown some merit in the utilisation of peritoneal dialysis, haemodialysis and thoracic lavage in particular when extracorporeal membrane oxygenation or cardiopulmonary bypass is not available.

Coma

Symptoms (as relayed by witnesses, family or friends)

➲ Seizure activity, altered level of consciousness, fever, chills, weakness, visual disturbance, memory loss, hallucinations, syncope, headache

Signs

➲ Hypotension, hypo- or hyperthermia, evidence of trauma, signs of underlying cause

➲ Further information may be obtained from use of the Glasgow Coma Scale

Ability	Score
Eye opening	
Spontaneous	4
To speech	3
To pain	2
No response	1
Best motor response	
To verbal command: obeys	6
To painful stimulus: localises pain	5
Flexion – withdrawal	4
Flexion – abnormal	3
Extension	2
No response	1
Best verbal response	
Oriented and converses	5
Disoriented and converses	4
Inappropriate words	3
Incomprehensible sounds	2
No response	1

Differentials

➲ Stroke
➲ Sepsis
➲ Hypo- or hyperglycaemia
➲ Hyponatraemia
➲ Brain tumour

- ⊃ Hypo- or hypercalcaemia
- ⊃ Hypothermia
- ⊃ Wernicke's encephalopathy

How to investigate and manage?

Investigations of choice include an arterial blood gas, full blood count, urea and electrolytes, glucose, liver function tests, coagulation profile, drug screen and blood cultures. Additional investigations include a CT or MRI head scan, a lumbar puncture if suspicious of meningitis and an electroencephalogram.

Management relies on treatment of the underlying cause.

SURGERY

Deep vein thrombosis

Symptoms
- ⊃ Limb pain, swelling, calf tenderness, skin redness, symptoms of a pulmonary embolism

Signs
- ⊃ Calf pain on foot dorsiflexion (Homans' sign), thrombophlebitis, signs of a pulmonary embolism

Differentials
- ⊃ Baker's cyst
- ⊃ Budd–Chiari syndrome
- ⊃ Cellulitis
- ⊃ Thrombophlebitis

How to investigate?

Investigations of choice include a D-dimer, which if positive should lead to imaging, depending on clinical probability, primarily via venous ultrasound. The Wells score helps to ascertain the clinical probability of a deep vein thrombosis or pulmonary embolism.

How to manage?

Suspected patients must be treated with therapeutic doses of low-molecular-weight heparin followed by warfarin, with a target international normalised ratio of 2.5. Low-molecular-weight heparin should only be considered instead of warfarin in cases of thrombosis secondary to malignancy. Treatment should be continued for up to 3 months in cases of the first episode of a deep vein thrombosis. Inferior vena cava filters are required in cases where there is a contraindication to anticoagulation, recurrent thromboembolism despite anticoagulation or active bleeding during treatment.

Deep Vein Thrombosis (DVT) Wells Score

Clinical feature	Points	Patient score
Active cancer (treatment on-going, within 6 months, or palliative)	1	
Paralysis, paresis or recent plaster immobilisation of the lower extremities	1	
Recently bedridden for 3 days or more or major surgery within 12 weeks requiring general or regional anaesthesia	1	
Localised tenderness along the distribution of the deep venous system	1	
Entire leg swollen	1	
Calf swelling at least 3 cm larger than asymptomatic side	1	
Pitting oedema confined to the symptomatic leg	1	
Collateral superficial veins (non-varicose)	1	
Previously documented DVT	1	
An alternative diagnosis is at least as likely as DVT	–2	
Clinical probability simplified score		
DVT *likely*	2 points or more	
DVT *unlikely*	1 point or lower	

Pulmonary Embolism (PE) Wells Score

Clinical feature	Points	Patient score
Clinical signs and symptoms of DVT (minimum of leg swelling and pain with palpation of the deep veins)	3	
An alternative diagnosis is less likely than PE	3	
Heart rate >100 beats per minute	1.5	
Immobilisation for more than 3 days or surgery in the previous 4 weeks	1.5	
Previous DVT or PE	1.5	
Haemoptysis	1	
Malignancy (on treatment, treated in the last 6 months, or palliative)	1	
Clinical probability simplified scores		
PE *likely*	More than 4 points	
PE *unlikely*	4 points or fewer	

Note: DVT, deep vein thrombosis

Acute appendicitis

Symptoms

⮞ Abdominal pain (central initially and then migrating to the right lower quadrant), vomiting, urinary symptoms, loss of appetite

Signs

⮞ Rebound tenderness, guarding, McBurney's point tenderness (tenderness one-third of the distance from the anterior superior iliac spine to the umbilicus), Rovsing's sign (right lower quadrant pain on palpation of the left lower quadrant)

Differentials

⮞ Abdominal abscess
⮞ Cholecystitis
⮞ Crohn's disease
⮞ Diverticular disease
⮞ Ectopic pregnancy
⮞ Gastroenteritis
⮞ Mesenteric ischaemia
⮞ Ovarian cyst
⮞ Pelvic inflammatory disease
⮞ Renal stones
⮞ Urinary tract infection

How to investigate?

Investigations of choice include a full blood count, urea and electrolytes, liver function tests, C-reactive protein and urinalysis. In addition, female patients should have a pregnancy test. Imaging of choice includes an abdominal ultrasound, computed tomography or MRI, of which computed tomography is the most sensitive and specific. MRI is reserved for cases of diagnostic difficulty.

How to manage?

Management relies on appropriate fluid resuscitation, surgical intervention and perioperative antibiotics (broad spectrum with Gram-negative and anaerobic cover) to reduce the risk of infection and abscess formation. Laparoscopic surgery is preferred, as it is associated with a lower risk of wound infection and hospital stay.

Small bowel obstruction

Symptoms

➲ Abdominal pain, vomiting, diarrhoea, constipation, fever

Signs

➲ Abdominal distension, hyperactive bowel sounds, fever, tachycardia, peritonism

Differentials

➲ Diabetic ketoacidosis
➲ Cholecystitis
➲ Constipation
➲ Diverticular disease
➲ Inflammatory bowel disease
➲ Mesenteric ischaemia

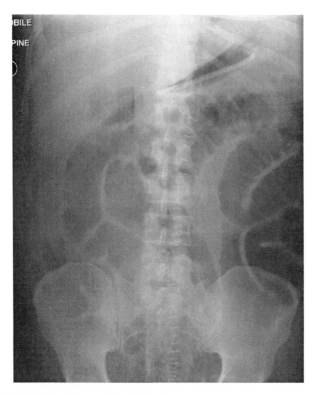

Abdominal X-ray demonstrating small bowel obstruction

How to investigate?

Investigations of choice include a full blood count, urea and electrolytes, lactate dehydrogenase, C-reactive protein, an abdominal X-ray (which will demonstrate small bowel dilatation and air fluid levels), a chest X-ray to exclude air under the diaphragm and an abdominal CT scan with contrast Gastrografin.

How to manage?

Patients should be kept nil by mouth with nasogastric tube placement and adequately fluid resuscitated with replacement of electrolytes that are deplete. Surgical intervention is generally employed in cases of complete small bowel obstruction with evidence of strangulation, perforation or in cases where resolution has not occurred within 48 hours.

Large bowel obstruction

Symptoms
- ⊃ Abdominal pain, nausea, vomiting, limited gas or bowel movement

Signs
- ⊃ Abdominal tenderness, fever, diminished bowel sounds, hyper-resonance on abdominal percussion, signs of peritonism in cases of perforation, evidence of inguinal and femoral hernias (often a cause of large bowel obstruction commonly missed!)

Differentials
- ⊃ Appendicitis
- ⊃ Diverticulitis
- ⊃ Pseudomembranous colitis
- ⊃ Small bowel obstruction
- ⊃ Toxic megacolon

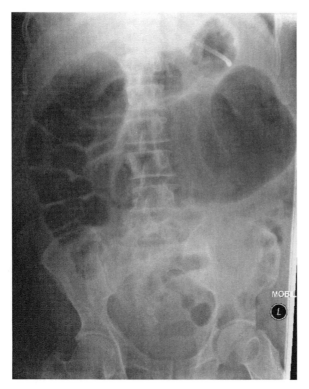

Abdominal X-ray demonstrating large bowel obstruction

How to investigate?

Investigations of choice include a full blood count, urea and electrolytes, CRP, lactate dehydrogenase, abdominal X-ray and CT scan of the abdomen with contrast. A flexible endoscopy may also be worthwhile in evaluation of left-sided colonic obstruction.

How to manage?

Patients should be kept nil by mouth with nasogastric tube placement with adequate fluid and electrolyte replacement. Management is usually conservative, with treatment of the underlying cause. However, in cases of limited resolution after 24–48 hours, surgical intervention is warranted. This is also true in cases of suspected or immediate perforation.

Acute mesenteric ischaemia

Symptoms
- ⊃ Pain, nausea, vomiting, diarrhoea or reduced ability to pass motion, bleeding per rectum, symptoms secondary to shock

Signs
- ⊃ Abdominal tenderness, peritonism, altered bowel sounds, signs of shock, atrial fibrillation (in cases of embolic acute mesenteric ischaemia)

Differentials
- ⊃ Abdominal abscess
- ⊃ Abdominal aortic aneurysm
- ⊃ Aortic dissection
- ⊃ Cholecystitis
- ⊃ Diverticulitis
- ⊃ Intestinal obstruction/perforation
- ⊃ Acute pancreatitis
- ⊃ Testicular torsion

How to investigate?

Investigations of choice include a full blood count, urea and electrolytes, C-reactive protein and lactate dehydrogenase. An abdominal X-ray is often warranted to exclude intestinal obstruction or perforation. More worthwhile investigations include an abdominal CT scan, mesenteric angiography and duplex ultrasound.

How to manage?

Management relies on adequate fluid and blood product resuscitation. Broad-spectrum antibiotics are key. Ensuring no contraindications to anticoagulation, patients should receive intravenous heparin with an activated partial thromboplastin time twice the normal value. Papaverine, a phosphodiesterase inhibitor, is used in cases of arterial embolic or non-occlusive disease. In cases of peritonism this is likely to imply bowel infarction, as opposed to ischaemia, and hence such individuals will require surgery. Embolectomy is the intervention of choice in acute mesenteric embolism. In cases of acute mesenteric ischaemia from arterial thrombosis due to atherosclerosis, a vascular bypass graft is essential. In cases of mesenteric venous thrombosis, patients should also be heparinised, and in view of main superior mesenteric vein or portal vein thrombosis, a thrombectomy is worthwhile. Use of thrombolytic agents such as alteplase have proven successful but are contraindicated when bowel infarction is suspected.

It is important to note that post-operatively such patients continue to require adequate fluid resuscitation, correction of renal failure and metabolic acidosis.

Acute cholecystitis

Symptoms

➲ Abdominal pain (right upper quadrant or epigastric with radiation to right shoulder), nausea and vomiting, fever

Signs

➲ Fever, tachycardia, hypotension, right upper quadrant or epigastric tenderness, Murphy's sign (inspiratory pause during palpation of right upper quadrant), palpable gall bladder, jaundice

Differentials

➲ Abdominal aortic aneurysm
➲ Acute mesenteric ischaemia
➲ Acute appendicitis
➲ Acute gastritis
➲ Acute pyelonephritis

How to investigate?

Investigations of choice include a full blood count, urea and electrolytes, serum amylase, liver function tests and C-reactive protein. Imaging of choice is an abdominal ultrasound scan; however, the gold standard is in the form of biliary scintigraphy (HIDA scan).

How to manage?

Management relies on patients being kept nil by mouth, with adequate fluid resuscitation and analgesia. Antibiotics of choice include cephalosporins such as cefuroxime and metronidazole. Surgical intervention is only required in less than a third of cases, either open or laparoscopically.

Acute diverticulitis

Symptoms
- ⮞ Abdominal pain (typically left lower quadrant pain), nausea, vomiting, constipation, diarrhoea, fever

Signs
- ⮞ Abdominal tenderness, palpable mass, peritonism, diminished bowel sounds

Differentials
- ⮞ Acute appendicitis
- ⮞ Acute cholecystitis
- ⮞ Intestinal obstruction
- ⮞ Acute gastritis
- ⮞ Mesenteric ischaemia
- ⮞ Acute pancreatitis
- ⮞ Acute pyelonephritis

How to investigate?
Blood investigations include a full blood count, urea and electrolytes and C-reactive protein. Imaging of choice primarily relies upon abdominal CT scanning.

How to manage?
Patients should be commenced on antibiotics, primarily ciprofloxacin and metronidazole. In cases of possible obstruction, patients should be kept nil by mouth, adequately fluid resuscitated and have a nasogastric tube inserted. Surgical intervention is required in cases of poor response to medical management, abscess or fistula formation, obstruction or perforation.

Acute renal calculi

Symptoms
- ⊃ Abdominal flank pain, blood in urine, nausea, vomiting

Signs
- ⊃ Tenderness in flanks, haematuria, reduced bowel sounds, inability to lie still

Differentials
- ⊃ Abdominal abscess
- ⊃ Acute glomerulonephritis
- ⊃ Appendicitis
- ⊃ Biliary colic
- ⊃ Cholecystitis
- ⊃ Diverticulitis
- ⊃ Duodenal ulcer
- ⊃ Peptic ulcer
- ⊃ Inflammatory bowel disease
- ⊃ Pancreatitis
- ⊃ Renal cell carcinoma
- ⊃ Urinary tract infection

How to investigate?
CT scanning is the main imaging tool of choice. A plain abdominal X-ray is useful initially in the case of radio opaque stones. Urine should be sent for microscopy and culture as well as screened for blood, calcium, oxalate, urate, sodium, phosphorous, citrate, magnesium and pH. A full blood count, urea and electrolytes, serum calcium, parathyroid hormone, phosphorus and uric acid level should be sent.

How to manage?
In view of pain, patients should be commenced on non-steroidal anti-inflammatory drugs such as diclofenac. However, such drugs should not be given in patients with a history of gastrointestinal bleeding or renal impairment. Patients should be appropriately fluid resuscitated and treated with anti-emetics as required. Antibiotics should be prescribed in cases of urinary tract infection and depending on sensitivities.

From an interventional perspective, management can involve shock wave lithotripsy in cases of renal calculi <2 cm, ureteroscopy and subsequent stone removal, as well as percutaneous nephrolithotomy. Percutaneous nephrolithotomy is the treatment of choice for stones >2 cm and in patients with abnormal anatomical renal structure.

Urgent intervention is generally required in cases of urinary tract obstruction, urosepsis, abdominal pain or vomiting and acute renal failure. Ureteral stones <5 mm typically pass spontaneously. Proximal ureteral stones <1 cm should be treated with shock wave lithotripsy. Ureteroscopy should be employed in cases of stones >1 cm and percutaneous nephrolithotomy should be instigated in cases of stones >2 cm. In cases of distal ureteral calculi, ureteroscopy or shock wave lithotripsy is often required for stones <1 cm. Ureteroscopy can also be used for stones >2 cm.

Acute pyelonephritis

Symptoms
- ➲ Fever, lower back pain, nausea, vomiting, blood in urine

Signs
- ➲ Fever, costovertebral angle tenderness

Differentials
- ➲ Appendicitis
- ➲ Prostatitis
- ➲ Pelvic inflammatory disease

How to investigate?
Investigations of choice involve urine for microscopy and culture as well as a full blood count, urea and electrolytes, C-reactive protein and blood cultures. The imaging modality of choice is computed tomography but an ultrasound may also be worthwhile.

How to manage?
Patients require appropriate analgesia in view of symptom control, in addition to fluid resuscitation and anti-emetics. Empirical antibiotic therapy is typically in the form of fluroquinolones, cephalosporins, penicillin or aminoglycosides. This should then be tailored according to sensitivities.

Testicular torsion

Symptoms

➲ Scrotal pain or swelling, inguinal swelling, nausea, vomiting, fever

Signs

➲ Scrotal tenderness or oedema, loss of cremasteric reflex, high testes position, negative Prehn's sign (physical lifting of testes does not relieve pain)

Differentials

➲ Appendicitis
➲ Scrotal trauma
➲ Testicular tumour
➲ Varicocele

How to investigate?

Investigations of choice include a urinalysis for nitrite and leucocytes to help exclude a urinary tract infection. A colour duplex ultrasound may also be useful.

How to manage?

The management of choice involves immediate scrotal exploration.

Abdominal aortic aneurysm

Symptoms
- Back, flank, abdominal or groin pain, nausea, vomiting, syncope

Signs
- Palpable abdominal aorta, signs of shock

Differentials
- Appendicitis
- Cholelithiasis
- Diverticular disease
- Peptic ulcer disease
- Small and large bowel obstruction
- Myocardial infarction
- Acute pancreatitis

How to investigate?

Imaging is the primary investigation of choice, with a focus on abdominal ultrasound and the main focus on abdominal computed tomography. Routine blood investigations should include a full blood count, urea and electrolytes and C-reactive protein.

How to manage?

Management comprises surgical intervention in all cases except generally in asymptomatic patients with an abdominal aortic aneurysm that is <5.5 cm. An alternative to open surgery is the use of percutaneously implanted stent grafts. From a medical perspective, patients should be commenced on beta blockers with control of risk factors such as hypercholesterolaemia.

Aortic dissection

Symptoms

- Chest pain, neck pain, abdominal pain, syncope, weakness, loss of sensation, hoarse voice (due to recurrent laryngeal nerve compression), symptoms allied to Horner's syndrome (ptosis, miosis, anhidrosis), dyspnoea, dysphagia

Signs

- Hyper- or hypotension, interarm blood pressure differential >20 mmHg, aortic regurgitation, signs of cardiac tamponade, signs of Horner's syndrome

Differentials

- Myocardial infarction
- Myocarditis
- Pleural effusion
- Pulmonary embolism

How to investigate?

Investigations of choice include a chest X-ray and ECG. Computed tomography and magnetic resonance angiography are the mainstay imaging modalities of choice. Blood investigations include a full blood count, urea and electrolytes, D-dimer and cardiac enzyme profile.

How to manage?

Patients are best managed with appropriate fluid resuscitation in the first instance. Beta blocker therapy can help to reduce blood pressure fluctuations. Management relies typically on the type of dissection. Type A, which affects the ascending aorta, requires urgent surgical input. Type B, which does not affect the ascending aorta, requires the use of medical management in the form of beta blockers and calcium channel blockers. In cases of complicated type B dissection, endovascular repair courtesy of stent grafting is required.

Acute limb ischaemia

Symptoms

➲ Pain in thigh, buttock or calf that is relieved by rest, numbness

Signs

➲ Absent pulses, atrophic skin, livedo reticularis, pallor, loss of sensation

Differentials

➲ Deep vein thrombosis
➲ Thrombophlebitis

How to investigate?

Blood investigations, primarily a full blood count and coagulation profile, are essential. Doppler flow assessment allows for true flow assessment, in addition to computed tomography or magnetic resonance angiography. Patients should also undergo ECG and echocardiogram assessment.

How to manage?

Management relies on endovascular revascularisation or open surgery. The former involves the use of unfractionated heparin, a multi-side-hole catheter that crosses the occlusion and subsequent delivery of thrombolytic agents. These commonly include alteplase, reteplase and tenecteplase. Surgery involves thromboembolectomy with a balloon catheter, bypass surgery and adjuncts such as endarterectomy, patch angioplasty and intraoperative thrombolysis. In the long term, patients require anticoagulation through warfarin or antiplatelet therapy.

Necrotising fasciitis

Symptoms
- Pain and tenderness in area of affected skin and muscle, fever

Signs
- Skin discolouration (redness, dusky purple, gangrenous, necrotic)

Differentials
- Cellulitis
- Gas gangrene
- Orchitis
- Acute epididymitis
- Testicular torsion
- Toxic shock syndrome

How to investigate?

Investigations of choice include a plain X-ray to assess for soft tissue air, in addition to a CT scan plus or minus an MRI. Blood investigations are also key and include a full blood count, serum glucose, urea and electrolytes and serum albumin, in addition to a coagulation profile and C-reactive protein. An arterial blood gas is required and will typically demonstrate a metabolic acidosis. An incisional biopsy can help to provide tissue samples for diagnostic purposes.

How to manage?

Management involves adequate fluid resuscitation with antibiotics depending on tissue sensitivity. Empirical treatment may involve penicillin, an aminoglycoside and clindamycin. Urgent surgical intervention is typically required with debridement.

Burns

Symptoms
- ⊃ Redness, pain, swelling, numbness, discharge, breathing difficulties (if involving airway)

Signs
- ⊃ Erythema, pyrexia, cardiorespiratory compromise, altered mental status

Differentials
- ⊃ Cellulitis
- ⊃ Toxic epidermal necrolysis

How to investigate?
Blood investigations comprise a full blood count, urea and electrolytes, C-reactive protein and erythrocyte sedimentation rate. If possible, a lesion biopsy should be performed and sent for microbiological assessment.

How to manage?
Minor burns should be cleaned with soap and water. Non-adhesive dressing padded by gauze is effective for superficial dermal burns. Dressings should be examined at 48 hours to reassess depth and the wound in general. Major burns should be irrigated with cool water for at least 20 minutes. Chemical burns may require longer periods of irrigation with input from toxicology specialists. Analgesia is essential in all cases and is governed courtesy of the World Health Organization's analgesic ladder. Facial burns require anaesthetic input as to whether patients may need intubation. Fluid resuscitation is paramount and is dependent on body weight and burn area. The Parkland formula is one of several that may be useful in this respect (amount of fluid required in 24 hours (mL) = 4 × Patient's weight (kg) × Percentage of body surface area involved in burns. Note the body surface area involved in burns is calculated by applying the rule of nines – 9% for each arm, 18% for each leg, 18% for the front of the torso, 18% for the back of the torso, and 9% for the head). Fluids of choice include Hartmann's solution. Normal saline should be avoided because of the risk of hyperchloraemic metabolic acidosis. Large burns benefit from colloid use.

Nutritional input is key because of increased energy consumption. Of course, it goes without saying that high dependency or intensive care unit and plastics input should be obtained from the onset.

References

Medicine

Adrogué HJ, Madias NE. Hyponatremia. *N Engl J Med*. 2000; **342**(21): 1581–9.

Asthma Guidelines. British Thoracic Society. 2012. www.brit-thoracic.org.uk/guide lines/asthma-guidelines.aspx

Balthazar EJ, Freeny PC, van Sonnenberg E. Imaging and intervention in acute pancreatitis. *Radiology*. 1994; **193**(2): 297–306.

Bauer MP, Kuijper EJ, van Dissel JT, *et al*. European Society of Clinical Microbiology and Infectious Diseases (ESCMID): treatment guidance document for *Clostridium difficile* infection (CDI). *Clin Microbiol Infect*. 2009; **15**(12): 1067–79.

Bederson JB, Connolly ES Jr, Batjer HH, *et al*. Guidelines for the management of aneurysmal subarachnoid hemorrhage: a statement for healthcare professionals from a special writing group of the Stroke Council, American Heart Association. *Stroke*. 2009; **40**(3): 994–1025.

Best Practice. *Bacterial Meningitis*. London: BMJ Evidence Centre. Available at: www.bestpractice.bmj.com/best-practice/monograph/539.html

Best Practice. *Malaria*. London: BMJ Evidence Centre. Available at: www.bestpractice.bmj.com/best-practice/monograph/161/basics/pathophysiology.html

Best Practice. *Spinal Cord Compression*. London: BMJ Evidence Centre. Available at: www.bestpractice.bmj.com/best-practice/monograph/1012.html

Best Practice. *Viral Meningitis*. London: BMJ Evidence Centre. Available at: www.bestpractice.bmj.com/best-practice/monograph/540.html

British Thoracic Society Standards of Care Committee Pulmonary Embolism Guideline Development Group. British Thoracic Society guidelines for the management of suspected acute pulmonary embolism. *Thorax*. 2003; **58**(6): 470–83.

Brown DJ, Brugger H, Boyd J, et al. Accidental hypothermia. *N Engl J Med*. 2012; **367**(20): 1930–8.

Coakley G, Matthews C, Field M, *et al*. BSR & BHPR, BOA, RCGP and BSAC guidelines for management of the hot swollen joint in adults. *Rheumatology (Oxford)*. 2006; **45**(8): 1039–41.

Dargan PI, Wallace CI, Jones AL. An evidence based flowchart to guide the management of acute salicylate (aspirin) overdose. *Emerg Med J.* 2002; **19**(3): 206–9.

Diabetes UK. *Management of the Hyperosmolar Hyperglycaemic State in Adults with Diabetes.* Available at: www.diabetes.nhs.uk

Diabetes UK. *The Management of Diabetic Ketoacidosis in Adults.* Available at: www.diabetes.org.uk

Dunn LT. Raised intracranial pressure. *J Neurol Neurosurg Psychiatry.* 2002; **73**(Suppl. 1): i23–7.

Gould FK, Denning DW, Elliott TS, *et al.* Guidelines for the diagnosis and antibiotic treatment of endocarditis in adults: a report of the Working Party of the British Society for Antimicrobial Chemotherapy. *J Antimicrob Chemother.* 2012; **67**(2): 269–89.

Howard SC, Jones DP, Pui CH. The tumour lysis syndrome. *N Engl J Med.* 2011; **364**(19): 1844–54.

Johnston SC, Rothwell PM, Nguyen-Huynh MN, *et al.* Validation and refinement of scores to predict very early stroke risk after transient ischemic attack. *Lancet.* 2007; **369**(9558): 283–92.

Lewington A, Kanagasundaram S. *Clinical Practice Guidelines: acute kidney injury.* Petersfield, Hampshire: UK Renal Association; 2011.

MacDuff A, Arnold A, Harvey J, *et al.* Management of spontaneous pneumothorax: British Thoracic Society Pleural Disease Guideline 2010. *Thorax.* 2010; **65**(Suppl. 2): ii18–31.

Maisch B, Seferović PM, Ristić AD, *et al.* Guidelines on the diagnosis and management of pericardial diseases executive summary; the Task Force on the Diagnosis and Management of Pericardial Diseases of the European Society of Cardiology. *Eur Heart J.* 2004; **25**(7): 587–610.

Medicines and Healthcare products Regulatory Agency (MHRA). *Paracetamol Overdose.* Available at: www.mhra.gov.uk

Mowat C, Cole A, Windsor A, *et al.* Guidelines for the management of inflammatory bowel disease in adults. *Gut.* 2011; **60**(5): 571–607.

National Institute for Health and Clinical Excellence (NICE). *The Epilepsies: the diagnosis and management of the epilepsies in adults and children in primary and secondary care; NICE guideline 137.* London: NICE; 2004. www.nice.org.uk/CG137

National Institute for Health and Clinical Excellence (NICE). *Atrial Fibrillation: NICE guideline 36.* London: NICE; 2006. www.nice.org.uk/CG36

National Institute for Health and Clinical Excellence (NICE). *Head Injury: triage, assessment, investigation and early management of head injury in infants, children and adults; NICE guideline 56.* London: NICE; 2007. www.nice.org.uk/cg56

National Institute for Health and Clinical Excellence (NICE). *Stroke: diagnosis and initial management of acute stroke and transient ischaemic attack (TIA); NICE guideline 68*. London: NICE; 2008. www.nice.org.uk/cg68

National Institute for Health and Clinical Excellence (NICE). *Chronic Obstructive Pulmonary Disease: NICE guideline 101*. London: NICE; 2010. http://guidance.nice.org.uk/cg101

National Institute for Health and Clinical Excellence (NICE). *Clopidogrel and Modified-Release Dipyridamole for the Prevention of Occlusive Vascular Events: NICE guideline 90*. London: NICE; 2010. www.nice.org.uk/ta210

National Institute for Health and Clinical Excellence (NICE). *Delirium: NICE guideline 103*. London: NICE; 2010. www.nice.org.uk/cg103

National Institute for Health and Clinical Excellence (NICE). *Acute Upper Gastrointestinal Bleeding: management; NICE guideline 141*. London: NICE; 2012. www.nice.org.uk/guidance/CG141

National Institute for Health and Clinical Excellence (NICE). *Neutropenic Sepsis: prevention and management of neutropenic sepsis in cancer patients; NICE guideline 151*. London: NICE; 2012. www.nice.org.uk/CG151

Nieminen MS, Böhm M, Cowie MR, *et al*. Executive summary of the guidelines on the diagnosis and treatment of acute heart failure: the Task Force on Acute Heart Failure of the European Society of Cardiology. *Eur Heart J*. 2005; **26**(4): 384–416.

Papini R. Management of burn injuries of various depths. *BMJ*. 2004; **329**(7458): 158–60.

Pleural Disease Guidelines. British Thoracic Society. 2010. www.brit-thoracic.org.uk/Guidelines/Pleural-Disease-Guidelines-2010.aspx

Pneumonia Guidelines. British Thoracic Society. 2009. www.brit-thoracic.org.uk/guidelines/pneumonia-guidelines.aspx

Polson J, Lee WM; American Association for the Study of Liver Disease. AASLD position paper: the management of acute liver failure. *Hepatology*. 2005; **41**(5): 1179–97.

Rees DC, Olujohungbe AD, Parker NE, *et al*. Guidelines for the management of the acute painful crisis in sickle cell disease. *Br J Haematol*. 2003; **120**(5): 744–52.

Reynolds HR, Hochman JS. Cardiogenic shock: current concepts and improving outcomes. *Circulation*. 2008; **117**(5): 686–97.

Scottish Intercollegiate Guidelines Network (SIGN). *Management of Acute Upper and Lower Gastrointestinal Bleeding: A national clinical guideline*. SIGN publication no. 105. Edinburgh, Scotland: SIGN; 2008.

Scottish Intercollegiate Guidelines Network (SIGN). *Acute Coronary Syndromes: A national clinical guideline*. SIGN publication no. 93 [2007; updated February 2013]. Edinburgh, Scotland: SIGN; 2013.

Stone MJ, Bogen SA. Evidence-based focused review of management of hyperviscosity syndrome. *Blood*. 2012; **119**(10): 2205–8.

Surviving Sepsis Campaign. *Guidelines*. Mount Prospect, IL: Society of Critical Care Medicine. Available at: www.survivingsepsis.org

Thwaites G. The management of suspected encephalitis. *BMJ*. 2012; **344**: e3489.

Uhl W, Warshaw A, Imrie C, *et al*. IAP guidelines for the surgical management of acute pancreatitis. *Pancreatology*. 2002; **2**(6): 565–73.

Varon J, Marik PE. Clinical review: the management of hypertensive crises. *Crit Care*. 2003; **7**(5): 374–84.

White HD, Chew DP. Acute myocardial infarction. *Lancet*. 2008; **372**(9638): 570–84.

Working Party of the British Society of Gastroenterology; Association of Surgeons of Great Britain and Ireland; Pancreatic Society of Great Britain and Ireland; *et al*. UK guidelines for the management of acute pancreatitis. *Gut*. 2005; **54**(Suppl. 3): iii1–9.

Surgery

Creager MA, Kaufman JA, Conte MS. Clinical practice: acute limb ischemia. *N Engl J Med*. 2012; **366**(23): 2198–206.

Hasham S, Matteucci P, Stanley PR, *et al*. Necrotising fasciitis. *BMJ*. 2005; **330**(7495): 830–3.

Humes DJ, Simpson J. Acute appendicitis. *BMJ*. 2006; **333**(7567): 530–4.

Indar AA, Beckingham IJ. Acute cholecystitis. *BMJ*. 2002; **325**(7365): 639–43.

Isselbacher EM. Thoracic and abdominal aortic aneurysms. *Circulation*. 2005; **111**(6): 816–28.

Jacobs DO. Clinical practice: diverticulitis. *N Engl J Med*. 2007; **357**(20): 2057–66.

Miller NL, Lingeman JE. Management of kidney stones. *BMJ*. 2007; **334**(7591): 468–72.

National Institute for Health and Care Excellence (NICE). *Venous Thromboembolic Diseases: Two-level Wells score; templates for deep vein thrombosis and pulmonary embolism*. London: NICE; 2013. Available at: http://guidance.nice.org.uk/CG144/TemplateWellsScore/doc/English

Oldenburg WA, Lau LL, Rodenberg TJ, *et al*. Acute mesenteric ischemia: a clinical review. *Arch Intern Med*. 2004; **164**(10): 1054–62.

Scottish Intercollegiate Guidelines Network (SIGN). *Prevention and Management of Venous Thromboembolism: A national clinical guideline*. SIGN publication no. 62. Edinburgh, Scotland: SIGN; 2010.

Somani BK, Watson G, Townell N. Testicular torsion. *BMJ*. 2010; **341**: c3213.

Thrumurthy SG, Karthikesalingam A, Patterson B, *et al*. The diagnosis and management of aortic dissection. *BMJ*. 2011; **344**: d8290.

Vallicelli C, Coccolini F, Catena F, *et al*. Small bowel emergency surgery: literature's review. *World J Emerg Surg*. 2011; **6**(1): 1.

Index

CT angiography, 8, 38; pulmonary, 23
CT head scan: and encephalitis, 42; and head injury, 43; and hypertensive crisis, 65; and hyperviscosity syndrome, 77; and hyponatraemia, 29; and hypothermia, 88; and malaria, 80; and meningitis, 40–1
CT myelograph, 34
Cullen's sign, 11
cyanosis: and anaphylaxis, 84; and ARDS, 20; and cardiogenic shock, 69; and COPD, 19; and DIC, 78; and heart failure, 63; and PE, 22; and pneumonia, 16; and respiratory failure, 21
cyclophosphamide, 76
cytology, 25, 69
cytomegalovirus, 41, 66

D-dimer, 23, 78, 92, 108
DC shock, 59
debridement, 110
dehydration: and aspirin overdose, 85; and *C. difficile*, 4; and diabetic ketoacidosis, 48; and gastroenteritis, 14; and hyperosmolar hyperglycaemic state, 49; and hyponatraemia, 29; and lower GI bleeding, 7
delirium, 38–9
delusions, 38
desmopressin, 76
dexamethasone, 52
dextrose, 14, 50, 52
diabetes: and atrial fibrillation, 54–5; and renal failure, 28
diabetic ketoacidosis, 48–9
diamorphine, 73
diarrhoea: and diverticulitis, 102; and gastroenteritis, 14; and IBD, 9; and lower GI bleeding, 7; and malaria, 79; and mesenteric ischaemia, 99; and pancreatitis, 11; and pneumonia, 16; and small bowel obstruction, 95; and thyroid storm, 50; watery, 4
diazepam, 40
DIC (disseminated intravascular coagulation), 78–9
diclofenac, 73, 103
digoxin, 55–7, 59
diltiazem, 59
diplopia: and stroke, 34; and subarachnoid haemorrhage, 37
dipyridamole, 37
discharge, 111
diuretics, 22, 31, 44, 63, 66
diverticular disease, 4, 8
diverticulitis, acute, 102
dizziness: and anaphylaxis, 83; and atrial fibrillation, 54; and bradycardia, 60; and heart block, 56; and hypothermia, 88; and renal failure, 28; and subarachnoid

haemorrhage, 37; and tachycardia, 58; and upper GI bleeding, 5
dobutamine: and cardiogenic shock, 70; and heart failure, 64; and neutropenic sepsis, 75
dopamine: and bradycardia, 61; and cardiogenic shock, 70; and heart failure, 64; and hypovolaemic shock, 82; and neutropenic sepsis, 75
Doppler flow assessment, 109
doxapram, 20
doxycycline, 80
dressings, 111
drowsiness, 44, 49
drug screen, 87, 90
DVT (deep vein thrombosis), 92–3; prophylaxis of, 21, 75
dysarthria, 34, 88
dysphagia, 5, 42, 108
dyspnoea: and acute coronary syndrome, 57; and anaphylaxis, 83; and aortic dissection, 108; and ARDS, 20; and aspirin overdose, 85; and asthma, 17; and atrial fibrillation, 54; and atrial flutter, 55; and bradycardia, 60; and cardiac tamponade, 68; and COPD, 19; and DIC, 78; and endocarditis, 65; and haemolytic anaemia, 75; and heart block, 56; and heart failure, 63; and hypothermia, 88; and myocarditis, 66; and neutropenic sepsis, 74; and PE, 22; and pericardial effusion, 68; and pericarditis, 67; and pleural effusion, 25; and pneumonia, 16; and pneumothorax, 23; and respiratory failure, 21; and sickle-cell disease, 72; and tachycardia, 58; and thyroid storm, 50; and tumour lysis syndrome, 77
dysrhythmias, 87

ECG (electrocardiogram): and acute coronary syndrome, 57; and anaphylaxis, 83–4; and aortic dissection, 108; and atrial fibrillation, 54; and atrial flutter, 55–6; and bradycardia, 60; and cardiac tamponade, 68; and cardiogenic shock, 70; and COPD, 20; and diabetic ketoacidosis, 48; and heart block, 56; and heart failure, 63; and hyperkalaemia, 30; and hyperosmolar hyperglycaemic state, 49; and hypertensive crisis, 64; and limb ischaemia, 109; and myocarditis, 66; and myxoedema crisis, 51; and pericardial effusion, 69; and pericarditis, 67; and renal failure, 28; and tachycardia, 58; and thyroid storm, 50
echocardiogram: and acute coronary syndrome, 57; and ARDS, 21; and atrial fibrillation, 54–5; and atrial flutter, 56; and cardiac arrest, 62; and cardiac tamponade, 68; and cardiogenic shock, 70;

echocardiogram (*cont.*) and endocarditis, 65; and heart failure, 63; and limb ischaemia, 109; and myocarditis, 66; and pericardial effusion, 69; and pericarditis, 67; and respiratory failure, 22; and stroke, 35

eclampsia, 35

ectopic pregnancy, 82

electroencephalogram, 39, 90

electrolytes: and abdominal aortic aneurysm, 107; and Addisonian crisis, 52; and anaphylaxis, 83; and aortic dissection, 108; and appendicitis, 94; and ARDS, 21; and aspirin overdose, 85; and asthma, 18; and atrial fibrillation, 54; and atrial flutter, 56; and bradycardia, 60–1; and burns, 111; and *C. difficile*, 4; and cardiac arrest, 62; and cardiac tamponade, 68; and cardiogenic shock, 70; and cholecystitis, 101; and coma, 90; and COPD, 20; and delirium, 39; and diabetic ketoacidosis, 48; and DIC, 78; and diverticulitis, 102; and encephalitis, 42; and endocarditis, 65; and gastroenteritis, 14; and heart block, 56; and heart failure, 63; and hypercalcaemia, 31; and hyperkalaemia, 30; and hyperosmolar hyperglycaemic state, 49; and hypertensive crisis, 64; and hypothermia, 88; and hypovolaemic shock, 82; and IBD, 10; and large bowel obstruction, 98; and lower GI bleeding, 8; and malaria, 79; and meningitis, 40–1; and mesenteric ischaemia, 99; and necrotising fasciitis, 110; and neutropenic sepsis, 74; and opioid overdose, 87; and paracetamol overdose, 86; and pericarditis, 67; and pneumonia, 16; and pyelonephritis, 105; and raised intracranial pressure, 44; and renal calculi, 103; and renal failure, 28–9; and respiratory failure, 22; and septic arthritis, 46; and small bowel obstruction, 96; and status epilepticus, 39; and tachycardia, 58–9; and thrombocytopenia, 76; and thyroid storm, 50; and TIA, 36; and tumour lysis syndrome, 77

embolectomy, 99

empyema, 25

encephalitis, 42

encephalopathy, 9, 29, 35

endarterectomy, 36–7, 109

endocarditis, infective, 65

endomyocardial biopsy, 66

endoscopic retrograde cholangiopancreatogram, 14

endoscopy, 6–7, 82, 98

endovascular coiling, 38

endovascular revascularisation, 109

Entamoeba, 14

enteral feeding, 14

Enterobacteriaceae, 66

enteroviruses, 41

eosinophil count, 18

eosinophilic pneumonia, 21

epidural abscess, 34

epigastric tenderness, 101

episcleritis, 9

epistaxis, and hyperviscosity syndrome, 77

Epstein–Barr virus, 66

erythema: and anaphylaxis, 83; and burns, 111; and septic arthritis, 46

erythema nodosum, 9

erythrocyte sedimentation rate: and burns, 111; and myocarditis, 66; and pericardial effusion, 69; and pericarditis, 67; and septic arthritis, 46

erythromycin, 14

Escherichia coli, 14, 41

European Carotid Surgery Trial criteria, 37

exercise tolerance, reduced, 56

extensor posturing, 43

exudates, 25, 64

eye pain, 37

eye twitching, 39

facial burns, 111

facial weakness, and TIA, 36

fainting, *see* syncope

fasciculations, 31

fatigue: and anaphylaxis, 84; and atrial flutter, 55; and cardiac tamponade, 68; and haemolytic anaemia, 75; and heart block, 56; and heart failure, 63; and malaria, 79; and myxoedema crisis, 51; and neutropenic sepsis, 74

femoral pulses, 64

fever: and aspirin overdose, 85; and *C. difficile*, 4; and cardiac tamponade, 68; and cholecystitis, 101; and coma, 89; and diverticulitis, 102; and encephalitis, 42; and endocarditis, 65; and gastroenteritis, 14; and hyperosmolar hyperglycaemic state, 49; and IBD, 9; and large bowel obstruction, 97; and lower GI bleeding, 7; and malaria, 79; and meningitis, 40–1; and myocarditis, 66; and necrotising fasciitis, 110; and neutropenic sepsis, 74; and pancreatitis, 11; and pericarditis, 67; and pleural effusion, 25; and pneumonia, 16; and pyelonephritis, 105; and renal failure, 28; and septic arthritis, 46; and sickle-cell disease, 72; and small bowel obstruction, 95; and stroke, 35; and testicular torsion, 106; and thyroid storm, 50

fibrinogen, 7, 78–9

finger clubbing, 65

fits, *see* seizures

flank pain, 107

haemodialysis, 9, 75, 85, 88
haemodynamic assessment, 70
haemodynamic compromise, 56
haemodynamic instability: and acute liver failure, 8; and Addisonian crisis, 52; and aspirin overdose, 85; and lower GI bleeding, 7; and paracetamol overdose, 86; and sickle-cell disease, 72; and thyroid storm, 50; and upper GI bleeding, 5
haemodynamic stability, 22
haemolytic anaemia, 75–6
haemoptysis, 16, 25, 72, 78, 93
haemorrhage, and hypertensive crisis, 64
haemotympanum, 43
hallucinations: and coma, 89; and delirium, 38; and status epilepticus, 39
haloperidol, 39, 73
Hartmann's solution, 111
head injury, 43
headache: and anaphylaxis, 83; and coma, 89; and encephalitis, 42; and endocarditis, 65; and gastroenteritis, 14; and head injury, 43; and hypercalcaemia, 31; and hypertensive crisis, 64; and hyperviscosity syndrome, 77; and hyponatraemia, 29; and malaria, 79; and meningitis, 40–1; and raised intracranial pressure, 44; and stroke, 34–5; thunderclap, 37
hearing loss: and head injury, 43; and renal failure, 28
heart block: and bradycardia, 61; complete, 56–7
heart failure: and atrial fibrillation, 54; congestive, 54; and endocarditis, 65; hypertensive, 35; and sickle-cell disease, 72; and upper GI bleeding, 6
heart rate, slow, 60
heart sound: diminished, 68; muffled, 68; third or fourth, 57, 63–4, 69
heart transplantation, 64
heartburn, 5
hemiparesis, 34, 37
hemisensory deficit, 34
hemofiltration, 75
heparin: and acute coronary syndrome, 57–8; and cardiogenic shock, 70; and diabetic ketoacidosis, 49; and DIC, 79; and DVT, 92; and limb ischaemia, 109; and mesenteric ischaemia, 99; and PE, 23; subcutaneous, 11
hepatitis, 9, 66
hepatomegaly, 63, 68
hepatosplenomegaly, 79
hernia, and large bowel obstruction, 97
herpes, 41–2
hoarseness, 84, 108
Homans' sign, 92
Horner's syndrome, 108

hydrocephalus, 38
hydrocortisone, 10–11, 52, 75, 84
hydroxychloroquine, 80
hydroxyzine, 73
hyper-reflexia, 31, 34, 50
hyperammonaemia, 29
hyperbilirubinaemia, 74
hypercalcaemia, 31; and renal failure, 29
hypercapnia, 18, 20–2
hypercholesterolaemia, 107
hyperglycaemia, 70, 74–5
hyperkalaemia, 30–1; and Addisonian crisis, 52; and cardiac arrest, 62; and hyperosmolar hyperglycaemic state, 49; and renal failure, 28–9
hyperlactataemia, 74
hypernatraemia, 29
hyperosmolar hyperglycaemic state, 49–50
hyperphosphataemia, 29
hyperpyrexia, 50
hypertension: and acute coronary syndrome, 57; and aortic dissection, 108; and atrial fibrillation, 54–5; and renal failure, 28; and stroke, 34; and subarachnoid haemorrhage, 37; and tumour lysis syndrome, 77
hypertensive crisis, 64–5
hyperthermia: and Addisonian crisis, 52; and coma, 89; and renal failure, 29
hyperthyroidism, and atrial flutter, 55
hyperuricaemia, 29
hyperventilation, 85
hyperviscosity syndrome, 77, 115
hypofibrinogenaemia, 79
hypoglycaemia, and myxoedema crisis, 51
hypokalaemia, 48–9, 62
hyponatraemia, 29–30; and Addisonian crisis, 52; and myxoedema crisis, 51; and subarachnoid haemorrhage, 38
hyporeflexia, 48, 88
hypotension: and acute coronary syndrome, 57; and anaphylaxis, 83; and aortic dissection, 108; and ARDS, 20; and atrial flutter, 55; and cardiac tamponade, 68; and cardiogenic shock, 69; and cholecystitis, 101; and coma, 89; and diabetic ketoacidosis, 48; and DIC, 78; and haemolytic anaemia, 75; and heart block, 56; and hyperosmolar hyperglycaemic state, 49; and hyponatraemia, 29; and hypothermia, 88; and hypovolaemic shock, 82; and IBD, 9; and myxoedema crisis, 51; and pericardial effusion, 68; and pneumothorax, 23; and sepsis, 74–5; and tachycardia, 58; and upper GI bleeding, 5
hypothermia, 88; and Addisonian crisis, 52; and coma, 89; and myxoedema crisis, 51; and renal failure, 29; and sepsis, 74; therapeutic, 62

hypovolaemia, 62
hypovolaemic shock, 82
hypoxia: and cardiac arrest, 62; and PE, 22; and respiratory failure, 21; and sepsis, 74

ibuprofen, 73
imipenem, 14
immune globulin, 75–6
immunosuppressive therapy, 76
incisional biopsy, 110
incontinence, 34
indigestion, 5
inferior vena cava filters, 92
inflammatory bowel disease (IBD), acute, 9–11
infliximab, 11
influenza, 66
inguinal swelling, 106
inotropes, 22
insulin: and cardiogenic shock, 70; and hyperosmolar hyperglycaemic state, 49; and neutropenic sepsis, 75; subcutaneous, 49
insulin–dextrose, 31
intra-aortic balloon counterpulsation, 64, 70
intracerebral haemorrhage, 35–6
intracranial mass, 38
intracranial pressure: monitoring, 44; raised, see raised intracranial pressure
intravenous fluids: and aspirin overdose, 85; and gastroenteritis, 14; and hyperosmolar hyperglycaemic state, 49–50; and hypothermia, 88; and sickle-cell disease, 73
intubation, 43, 63, 111
ipratropium bromide, 18
ischaemic stroke, 35–8, 54
isoprenaline, 61
itching, 83

Janeway lesions, 65
jaundice: and acute liver failure, 8; and cholecystitis, 101; and DIC, 78; and haemolytic anaemia, 75; and malaria, 79; and paracetamol overdose, 86
jaw discomfort, 57
joint deformities, 72
joint discomfort, 76
joint pain: and endocarditis, 65; and malaria, 79; and renal failure, 28; and septic arthritis, 46
joint position, and cord compression, 34
joint swelling, 9, 46

Kernig's sign, 40
ketone measurement, 48–9
kidney injury, acute, 28–9

labetalol, 65
lactate dehydrogenase: and haemolytic

anaemia, 75; and large bowel obstruction, 98; and malaria, 79; and mesenteric ischaemia, 99; and pancreatitis, 12; and pericardial effusion, 69; and pericarditis, 67; and pleural effusion, 25; and small bowel obstruction, 96; and tumour lysis syndrome, 77
lactate measurement, 8, 49
lactulose, 9, 73
laparoscopic surgery, 94
large bowel obstruction, 98
laxatives, 73
left ventricular ejection fraction, 66
leg swelling, 93
leg ulcers, 75
Legionella, 16
lesion biopsy, 111
lethargy, 8, 49, 51, 77
leukocytosis, 74
Lewy body dementia, 39
light-headedness: and bradycardia, 60; and hypovolaemic shock, 82; and pericardial effusion, 68; and tachycardia, 58
Light's criteria, 25
limb ischaemia, acute, 109
limb jerking, 39
limb pain, 92
limb weakness: and cord compression, 34; and hyperkalaemia, 30; and hypertensive crisis, 64; and hyperviscosity syndrome, 77; and sickle-cell disease, 72
lip smacking, 39
lipase, 12
lipid studies, 12, 36
Listeria, 41
livedo reticularis, 28, 109
liver disease, chronic, 5
liver failure, acute, 8–9
liver function tests: and acute liver failure, 8; and appendicitis, 94; and ARDS, 21; and aspirin overdose, 85; and cardiogenic shock, 70; and cholecystitis, 101; and coma, 90; and delirium, 39; and head injury, 43; and heart failure, 63; and malaria, 79; and neutropenic sepsis, 74; and opioid overdose, 87; and pancreatitis, 12; and paracetamol overdose, 86; and pneumonia, 16; and septic arthritis, 46; and sickle-cell disease, 72; and status epilepticus, 39; and upper GI bleeding, 7
lobe consolidation, 17
lorazepam, 40
lower GI (gastrointestinal) bleeding, 7–8
Lugol's iodine, 50
lumbar puncture, 38–42, 90
lung expansion, asymmetrical, 23
lung scanning, isotope, 23

pulmonary artery catheterisation, 70
pulmonary embolism (PE), 22–3; and DVT, 92
pulmonary function tests, 22
pulmonary oedema: acute, 22; and acute coronary syndrome, 57; and bradycardia, 60; cardiogenic, 21; and hyperviscosity syndrome, 77; and hypovolaemic shock, 82; and malaria, 79; and tumour lysis syndrome, 77
pulse: absent, 109; diminished volume, 63; irregular, 54; rapid, 58
pulse oximetry, 84
pulsus paradoxus, 68
pupillary abnormalities, 43–4
pupils, fixed, 88
purpura, and thrombocytopenia, 76
pyelonephritis, acute, 105
pyoderma gangrenosum, 9
pyrexia, 111

quinine, 80

raised intracranial pressure, 44; and lumbar puncture, 38; and mannitol, 9
rash: and meningitis, 40–1; and myocarditis, 66; and neutropenic sepsis, 74; and renal failure, 28
rate control, 54–5
recombinant human activated protein C, 79
rectal bleeding, 14, 99
rectal examination, 7
reflexes: brisk, 41; slow relaxing, 51
renal artery bruit, 64
renal calculi, acute, 103–4
renal failure: acute, 28–9; correction of, 100; and liver failure, 9; and malaria, 79; and renal calculi, 104
renal function tests, 51
renal insufficiency, 30
renal profile, 7–8, 43, 69, 77
renal replacement, 28–9, 75
respiratory acidosis, 18
respiratory alkalosis, 85
respiratory arrest, 18
respiratory depression, 73
respiratory failure, 21–2
respiratory rate, reduced, 87
reteplase, 109
reticulocyte count, 72, 79
retinal haemorrhage, 76
rhythm control, 54–5
rigors, 46
rituximab, 76
Rockall scoring, 5–7
Roth's spots, 65

salbutamol, 31
salicylate levels, 85
saline: and burns, 111; and gastroenteritis, 14; hypertonic, 38; and myxoedema crisis, 51
saline replacement, 30, 52
Salmonella, 14
scleral icterus, 72
scrotal pain, 106
seizures: and aspirin overdose, 85; and coma, 89; and encephalitis, 42; and hyperosmolar hyperglycaemic state, 49; and hyperviscosity syndrome, 77; and hyponatraemia, 29; and malaria, 79; and meningitis, 41; post-traumatic, 43; and raised intracranial pressure, 44; and respiratory failure, 21; and subarachnoid haemorrhage, 37–8; and thyroid storm, 50; and tumour lysis syndrome, 77
senna, 73
sensation, loss of, 34, 43, 108–9
sensory loss, 29
sepsis: and encephalopathy, 9; and endocarditis, 66; and pneumonia, 16; recognising and managing, 74–5; see also neuropenic sepsis
septic arthritis, 46
serum albumin, 12, 110
serum amylase, 12, 72, 101
serum ANA, 28
serum bilirubin, 75
serum calcium, 12, 30, 39, 103
serum cholesterol, 12
serum cortisol, 29, 52
serum glucose: and Addisonian crisis, 52; and aspirin overdose, 85; and bradycardia, 60; and hypothermia, 88; and hypovolaemic shock, 82; and malaria, 79; and myxoedema crisis, 51; and necrotising fasciitis, 110; and pancreatitis, 12; and paracetamol overdose, 86; and status epilepticus, 39
serum haptoglobins, 75
serum lactate, 4, 70, 74
serum magnesium, 39
serum osmolality, 29, 49
serum sodium, 49
serum urea, 29, 52
serum viscosity, 77
Shigella, 14
shock: and bradycardia, 61; and mesenteric ischaemia, 99; and tachycardia, 59
shock wave lithotripsy, 103–4
SIADH (syndrome of inappropriate antidiuretic hormone secretion), 30
sickle-cell disease, 72–3
sickle-cell screen, 75
sigmoidoscopy, 4, 10, 14
silver wiring, 64
sinus tachycardia, 58
skin: atrophic, 109; clammy, 57, 82, 84; dry, 51; pain and tenderness in, 110; thickened, 51

thyroid function tests: and atrial fibrillation, 54; and atrial flutter, 56; and bradycardia, 60; and cardiac arrest, 62; and delirium, 39; and hyponatraemia, 29; and tachycardia, 58; and thyroid storm, 50
thyroid-stimulating hormone, 51
thyroid storm, 50
thyrotoxicosis, 50
tinnitus, and aspirin overdose, 85
tone, increased, 39
torsade de pointes, 59
toxic megacolon, 4, 10–11
toxicology screen, 9, 39, 62
tracheal deviation, 16, 23, 25
transcutaneous pacing, 57, 61
transient ischaemic attack (TIA), 36–7; and atrial fibrillation, 54
transvenous pacing, 61
trauma, and coma, 89
tremor, 43, 85
tricuspid regurgitation, 63
troponin: and acute coronary syndrome, 57; and atrial fibrillation, 54; and myocarditis, 66; and pericarditis, 67
Truelove criteria, 11
tumour-associated oedema, 34
tumour lysis syndrome, 77–8; and renal failure, 29

ulcerative colitis, 4, 11
ulcers, 74
ultrafiltration, 64
ultrasound: carotid, 36; duplex, 99, 106; and pyelonephritis, 105; renal, 28; transcranial, 35; venous, 92; see also abdominal ultrasound
upper gastrointestinal (GI) bleeding, 5–7
urea: and abdominal aortic aneurysm, 107; and anaphylaxis, 83; and aortic dissection, 108; and appendicitis, 94; and ARDS, 21; and aspirin overdose, 85; and asthma, 18; and atrial fibrillation, 54; and atrial flutter, 56; and bradycardia, 60; and burns, 111; and *C. difficile*, 4; and cardiac arrest, 62; and cardiac tamponade, 68; and cardiogenic shock, 70; and cholecystitis, 101; and coma, 90; and COPD, 20; and delirium, 39; and diabetic ketoacidosis, 48; and DIC, 78; and diverticulitis, 102; and encephalitis, 42; and endocarditis, 65; and gastroenteritis, 14; and heart block, 56; and heart failure, 63; and hypercalcaemia, 31; and hyperkalaemia, 30; and hyperosmolar hyperglycaemic state, 49; and hypertensive crisis, 64; and hypothermia, 88; and hypovolaemic shock, 82; and IBD, 10; and large bowel obstruction, 98; and lower GI bleeding, 8; and malaria, 79; and meningitis, 40–1;

and mesenteric ischaemia, 99; and necrotising fasciitis, 110; and neutropenic sepsis, 74; and opioid overdose, 87; and pancreatitis, 12; and paracetamol overdose, 86; and pericarditis, 67; and pneumonia, 16; and pyelonephritis, 105; and raised intracranial pressure, 44; and renal calculi, 103; and renal failure, 28; and respiratory failure, 22; and septic arthritis, 46; and small bowel obstruction, 96; and status epilepticus, 39; and tachycardia, 58; and thrombocytopenia, 76; and thyroid storm, 50; and TIA, 36
urea cycle defects, 29
ureteroscopy, 103–4
uric acid level, 103
urinalysis, 30, 64, 82, 94, 106
urinary alkalinisation, 85
urinary frequency, increasing, 31, 48–9
urinary hesitancy, 28, 34
urinary screen, 16, 39, 65
urinary sodium, 28–9
urinary symptoms: and appendicitis, 94; and tumour lysis syndrome, 77
urinary tract infection, 103, 106
urinary tract obstruction, 104
urinary urgency, 9, 28
urine: blood in, 28, 103, 105; dark, 75
urine cultures, 72
urine electrolytes, 28
urine microscopy, 48–9, 103, 105
urine osmolality, 28–30
urine output, 28–9, 49, 69, 74
urine pH, 77
urticaria, 83

vagal manoeuvres, 59
valve disease, 55
valvular failure, acute, 64
vancomycin, 4, 34, 40, 66
variceal bleeds, 7
vascular bypass graft, 99
vascular disease, and atrial fibrillation, 54–5
vasodilator therapy, 63
vasopressors, 70, 75, 82
venous pressure, elevated, 63, 68–9
ventilation: and cardiac arrest, 62; and head injury, 43; mechanical, 18, 22, 63; non-invasive, 20; positive pressure, 21–2
ventilatory support, 18, 63
ventricular fibrillation, 62
ventricular function, impaired, 55
ventricular pause, 61
ventricular septal defects, 64
ventricular tachycardia, 59, 62
vertigo, 34
vision, double, see diplopia
visual disturbance: and aspirin overdose, 85; and coma, 89; and hyperosmolar hyperglycaemic state, 49; and

hypertensive crisis, 64; and status epilepticus, 39
visual field defects, 34, 36, 44
visual loss: and hyperviscosity syndrome, 77; and raised intracranial pressure, 44; and sickle-cell disease, 72; and stroke, 34; and subarachnoid haemorrhage, 37
vitamin D, 31
vitamin K, 9
vomit, coffee-ground, 5
vomiting: and abdominal aortic aneurysm, 107; and acute coronary syndrome, 57; and Addisonian crisis, 52; and anaphylaxis, 83; and appendicitis, 94; and aspirin overdose, 85; and cardiogenic shock, 69; and cholecystitis, 101; and diabetic ketoacidosis, 48; and diverticulitis, 102; and encephalitis, 42; and gastroenteritis, 14; and head injury, 43; and heart failure, 63; and hypercalcaemia, 31; and IBD, 9; and large bowel obstruction, 97; and malaria, 79; and meningitis, 41; and mesenteric ischaemia, 99; and pancreatitis, 11; and paracetamol overdose, 86; and pyelonephritis, 105; and raised intracranial pressure, 44; and renal calculi, 103–4; and small bowel obstruction, 95; and subarachnoid haemorrhage, 37; and testicular torsion, 106; and thyroid storm, 50; and tumour lysis syndrome, 77
von Willebrand's disease, 76

warfarin, 7, 55, 92, 109
weakness: and aortic dissection, 108; and coma, 89; and delirium, 38; and diabetic ketoacidosis, 48; and DIC, 78; and encephalitis, 42; and haemolytic anaemia, 75; and hypercalcaemia, 31; and hyperkalaemia, 30; and hyperosmolar hyperglycaemic state, 49; and hyperviscosity syndrome, 77; and hypovolaemic shock, 82; and neutropenic sepsis, 74; and status epilepticus, 39; and stroke, 34; and subarachnoid haemorrhage, 37; and TIA, 36; and tumour lysis syndrome, 77; and upper GI bleeding, 5
Wegener's granulomatosis, 28
weight gain, and myxoedema crisis, 51
weight loss: and cardiac tamponade, 68; and diabetic ketoacidosis, 48; and endocarditis, 65; and hyperosmolar hyperglycaemic state, 49; and IBD, 9; and lower GI bleeding, 7; and pleural effusion, 25; and thyroid storm, 50; and upper GI bleeding, 5
Wells score, 92–3
wheeze, 17, 19, 63, 83–4
white blood cell count, 12
Witts' criteria, 11

X-ray: plain, 110; *see also* abdominal X-ray; chest X-ray; spinal X-ray
xanthochromia, 38

CPD with Radcliffe

You can now use a selection of our books to achieve CPD (Continuing Professional Development) points through directed reading.

We provide a free online form and downloadable certificate for your appraisal portfolio. Look for the CPD logo and register with us at: www.radcliffehealth.com/cpd

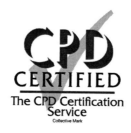

CERTIFIED
The CPD Certification
Service
Collective Mark